Ophthalmology Illness Scripts

Marta Ugarte

Ophthalmology Illness Scripts

Thinking like an Eye Doctor

Springer

Marta Ugarte
Faculty of Biology, Medicine and Health
University of Manchester
Manchester Royal Eye Hospital
Manchester University NHS Foundation Trust
Manchester, UK

ISBN 978-3-032-31007-1 ISBN 978-3-032-31008-8 (eBook)
https://doi.org/10.1007/978-3-032-31008-8

This Springer imprint is published by the registered company Springer Nature Switzerland AG
The registered company address is: Gewerbestrasse 11, 6330 Cham, Switzerland

To all undergraduates and postgraduates studying clinical ophthalmology, past, present and future

Preface

This book provides 50 ophthalmology illness scripts to prepare clinical ophthalmology students to think like eye doctors. It has been prepared based on 25-year experience working as an eye doctor. Solving clinical problems requires basic science and clinical knowledge, as well as the ability to compare different conditions. These illness scripts will guide clinical ophthalmology students while gaining clinical experience and developing their proficiency in clinical reasoning. These illness scripts will form the fundamental knowledge structures, which learners will be able to update and refine with each new patient encounter, throughout their careers.

The experience-based fine-tuning of these illness scripts will transform a student's knowledge-based thinking into an expert's experience-based clinical reasoning.

Manchester, UK Marta Ugarte

Competing Interests The author has no competing interests to declare that are relevant to the content of this manuscript.

Contents

Abbreviations

ACE	Angiotensin-converting enzyme
AF	Atrial fibrillation
AION	Anterior ischaemic optic neuropathy
ARMS2	Age-related maculopathy susceptibility 2 gene
ATP	Adenosine triphosphate
AV	Arteriovenous
BMI	Body mass index
BP	Blood pressure
BRB	Blood retinal barrier
CF	Counting fingers
CFH	Complement factor H
Ch	*Chlamydia*
CMV	Cytomegalovirus
CNS	Central nervous system
CRP	C reactive proteins
CRVO	Central retinal vein occlusion
CT	Computerized tomography
CYP1B1	Cytochrome P450 Family 1 Subfamily B Member 1
DNA	Deoxyribonucleic acid
ECG	Electrocardiogram
ENT	Ear nose and throat
ESR	Erythrocyte sedimentation rate
FB	Foreign body
FBC	Full blood count
FDA	Food and Drug Administration
GCA	Giant cell arteritis

HbA1c	Haemoglobin A1c
HLA	Human leukocyte antigen
HLAB27	Human leukocyte antigen B27
HSV	Herpes simplex virus
HZO	Herpes zoster ophthalmicus
ICG	Indocyanine green
IL6	Interleukin 6
IL8	Interleukin 8
IOL	Intraocular lens implant
IOP	Intraocular pressure
IRF	Intraretinal fluid
IRMA	Intraretinal microvascular abnormalities
IV	Intravenous
LP	Lumbar puncture
LT	Leukotriend
MGO	Myelin oligodendrocyte glycoprotein
MRA	Magnetic resonance angiography
MRI	Magnetic resonance imaging
MS	Multiple sclerosis
MT-ND1	Mitochondrial NADH dehydrogenase 1 protein gene
MT-ND4	Mitochondrial NADH dehydrogenase 4 protein gene
MT-ND6	Mitochondrial NADH dehydrogenase 6 protein gene
MYOC	Myocilin gene
NICE	National Institute for Health and Care Excellence
NMO	Neuromyelitis optica
NPDR	Non-proliferative diabetic retinopathy
NVD	Neovascularization at the optic disc
NVE	Neovascularization elsewhere in the retina
OCT	Optical coherence tomography
PCR	Polymerase chain reaction
PDR	Proliferative diabetic retinopathy
PED	Pigment epithelium detachment
PG	Prostaglandin
PHMB	Poly hexamethylene biguanide
PMN	Polymorphonuclear
PMR	Polymyalgia rheumatica
PRP	Panretinal photocoagulation
PRPH2	Peripherin 2 gene

RAPD	Relative afferent pupillary defect
RGC	Retinal ganglion cell
RNA	Ribonucleic acid
RPE	Retinal pigment epithelium
SLE	Systemic lupus erythematosus
SPEEs	Superficial punctate epitheliopathy
SRF	Subretinal fluid
SRS	Subretinal space
STD	Sexually transmitted disease
TB	Tuberculosis
Th17	T helper 17 cell
TIA	Transient ischaemic attack
TIMP3	Tissue inhibitor metalloprotease 3
URTI	Upper respiratory tract infection
UV	Ultraviolet
VEGF	Vascular endothelial growth factor
VZV	Varicella zoster virus
WDR36	WD Repeat Domain 36 gene

1 Principles of Illness Scripts and Their Use in Clinical Reasoning

An illness script is a comprehensive framework with organized knowledge about a specific disease [1]. The components of an illness script include the following: (a) cause (fault), (b) risk factors (enablers), (c) mechanisms (pathophysiology), (d) consequences (symptoms, signs, complications), (e) natural history and prognosis, (f) investigations and (g) management (treatment) of the disease. Illness scripts are dynamic and versatile structures. They are constantly developed and refined with experience with patients and learning.

The use of illness scripts facilitates clinical reasoning and diagnosis by contrasting and comparing different diseases and a particular patient's presentation. One of the primary functions of comparing illness scripts is to identify distinguishing features to narrow down a diagnosis. These are features, which are specific or highly suggestive of one diagnosis. Their presence or absence has a high predictive value for a particular diagnosis.

In this book, we provide 50 illness scripts of ophthalmology conditions highlighting distinguishing features and red flags. The latter are specific warning signs or symptoms suggesting a potentially serious underlying pathology, which requires immediate investigation and/or urgent specialist referral. The use of these structured illness scripts will guide readers and learners to build and apply their knowledge and develop robust clinical reasoning skills.

M. Ugarte, *Ophthalmology Illness Scripts*,
https://doi.org/10.1007/978-3-032-31008-8_1

Reference

1. Lubarsky S, Dory V, Audétat MC, Custers E, Charlin B. Using script theory to cultivate illness script formation and clinical reasoning in health professions education. Can Med Educ J. 2015;6(2):e61–70.

Blepharitis

2

Blepharitis is a common condition with chronic bilateral eyelid inflammation leading to symptoms of red, swollen and irritated eyelids (Figs. 2.1, 2.2, 2.3, and 2.4). There are two types, anterior (Fig. 2.1) and posterior blepharitis (Fig. 2.3), which may coexist in the same eyelid.

The illness scripts in Figs. 2.2 and 2.4, and Table 2.1, describe and compare the elements of anterior and posterior blepharitis.

M. Ugarte, *Ophthalmology Illness Scripts*,
https://doi.org/10.1007/978-3-032-31008-8_2

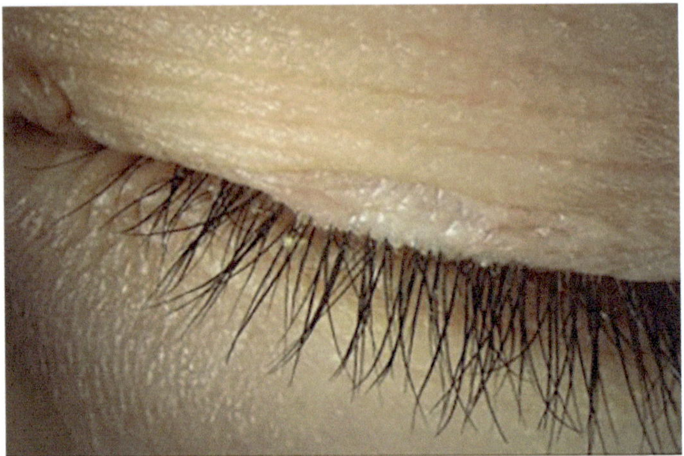

SIGNS

- Flakes, crusts around eyelashes roots
- Red, swollen, greasy eyelids
- Some cases: eyelashes madarosis or trichiasis
- Unstable precorneal tear film

Fig. 2.1 Anterior blepharitis

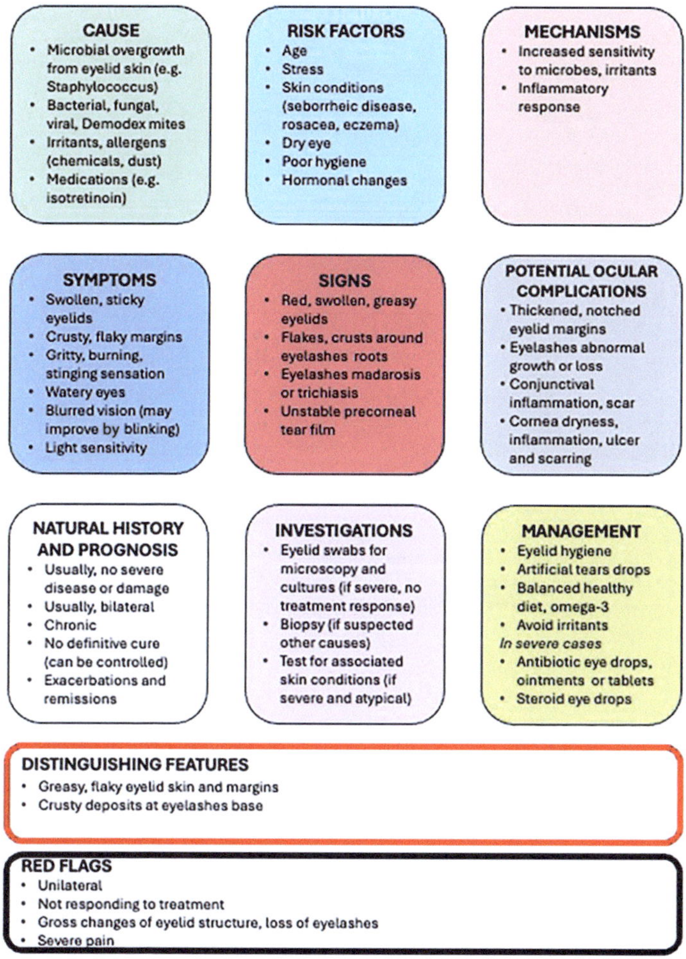

Fig. 2.2 Anterior blepharitis illness script (illness script 1)

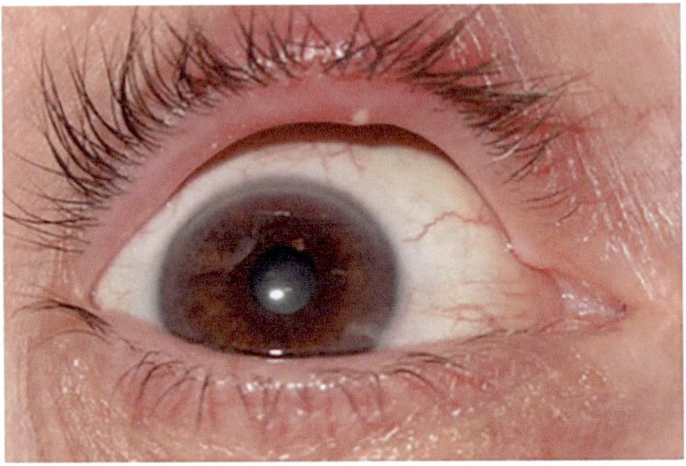

SIGNS

- Meibomian glands capped, dilated, obstructed
- Red, swollen eyelids
- Unstable precorneal tear film

Fig. 2.3 Posterior blepharitis

CAUSE
- Meibomian gland dysfunction

RISK FACTORS
- Skin conditions (e.g. seborrhoeic dermatitis)
- Microbial overgrowth on the eyelids
- Contact lens wear
- Eye makeup
- Hormonal changes
- Certain medications and systemic disease

MECHANISMS
- Meibomian gland dysfunction
- Trapping of meibum
- Deficient tears oily layer
- Tear film disruption
- Chronic inflammation

SYMPTOMS
- Red, swollen, greasy, sticky eyelids
- Crusty, flaky deposits at lid margin
- Gritty, burning, itching sensation
- Blurred vision (improves by blinking)
- Light sensitivity

SIGNS
- Meibomian glands capped, dilated, obstructed
- Red, swollen eyelids
- Unstable precorneal tear film

POTENTIAL OCULAR COMPLICATIONS
- Chalazion
- Changes in eyelid margin +/- eyelashes
- Conjunctival inflammation, scar
- Cornea dryness, inflammation, infection, scar
- Infection and spread

NATURAL HISTORY AND PROGNOSIS
- Usually, not severe
- Usually, bilateral
- Chronic
- Periods of exacerbation and remission

INVESTIGATIONS
- Eyelid swabs for microscopy, cultures or PCR (if atypical, no treatment response)
- Biopsy (if malignancy suspected)
- Check for associated skin conditions (in severe, atypical)

MANAGEMENT
- Eyelid hygiene
- Warm compresses
- Eyelid massage
- Lubricant eye drops
- Balanced diet, Omega-3

If severe:
- Antibiotics eye drops, ointments or tablets
- Steroid drops

DISTINGUISHING FEATURES
- Inflammation of the posterior lid margin +/- telangiectasias
- Meibomian glands dilated, obstructed, capped; with thickened, waxy, white/yellow secretions

RED FLAGS
- Unilateral
- Extreme redness and pain
- Reduced vision

Not responding to treatment
Changes in eyelids shape +/- eyelashes loss
Photophobia

Fig. 2.4 Posterior blepharitis illness script (illness script 2)

Table 2.1 Anterior and posterior blepharitis illness scripts comparison

	Anterior blepharitis	Posterior blepharitis
Cause	Microbial overgrowth from eyelid skin (e.g. *Staphylococcus*) bacterial, fungal, viral, Demodex mites Irritants, allergens (chemicals, dust) Medications (e.g. isotretinoin)	Meibomian gland dysfunction
Risk factors	Age Stress Dry eye Poor hygiene Skin conditions (seborrhoeic disorders, rosacea, eczema) Hormonal changes	Skin conditions (seborrheic dermatitis, rosacea, psoriasis) Bacterial overgrowth on the eyelids Demodex mites (microscopic) infesting eyelids Viral infections (e.g. herpes or shingles) Eye makeup irritation or poor removal Contact lens wear Hormonal changes Certain medication (e.g. anticholinergics, antihistamines) Systemic conditions (e.g. diabetes)
Mechanisms and pathogenesis	Increased sensitivity to bacterial overgrowth on eyelid skin Inflammatory response	Meibomian gland obstruction, dysfunction, trapping oily substance (meibum) Tear film disruption (deficient oily layer of tears) Chronic inflammation

(continued)

Table 2.1 (continued)

	Anterior blepharitis	Posterior blepharitis
Symptoms	Red and swollen eyelids Crusty, flaky dandruff at the base of the eyelashes Sticky eyelids (specially upon waking up) Gritty, burning, stinging sensation in the eyes Blurred vision (temporary), may improve with blinking Watery eyes Light sensitivity Wearing contact lenses may be uncomfortable	Irritation, redness and swelling of the eyelids Gritty, burning, itching feeling Crusty flaky deposits at the eyelashes Greasy, sticky eyelids Blurred vision (improving with blinking) Light sensitivity Dry eye symptoms
Signs	Red, swollen, greasy eyelid margins Flakes or crusts around the roots of the eyelashes Eyelash may fall out or grow in the wrong direction Unstable precorneal tear film	Oil glands capped, dilated, obstructed Unstable precorneal tear film
Natural history and prognosis	Chronic No definitive cure (but can be controlled) For most people, no severe disease or lasting eye damage Periods of exacerbation and remission Usually, bilateral	Chronic Periods of exacerbation and remission Usually, bilateral
Investigations	Eyelid swabs for microscopy and cultures (if very severe, not responding to treatment) Eyelid biopsy (if suspected other causes) Check for associated skin conditions	Eyelid swabs for microscopy, cultures or PCR (if atypical, not responding to treatment) Biopsy (if malignancy suspected) Check for associated skin conditions

(continued)

Table 2.1 (continued)

	Anterior blepharitis	Posterior blepharitis
Complications	Thickened, notched eyelid margins Eyelashes misdirection, abnormal growth, loss Conjunctival inflammation and scarring Cornea inflammation, ulcer and scarring Dry eye	Eyelid cyst (chalazion) Changes in eyelid margin and eyelashes Conjunctival inflammation and scarring Cornea inflammation Dry eye
Management	Eyelid hygiene with mild, warm solution, daily Artificial tears eye drops Antibiotic (e.g. chloramphenicol) eye drops or ointments, steroid eye drops, oral antibiotics (doxycycline) (severe cases) Avoid irritants Balanced healthy diet, consider omega-3 intake	Daily eyelid hygiene (mild, warm solution) Warm compresses Eyelid massage Lubricant eye drops Antibiotics eye drops or ointments (e.g. chloramphenicol) for severe cases Oral antibiotics (e.g. Doxycycline) for 6–12 weeks to reduce inflammation Omega-3 supplements can be considered Steroid drops for severe inflammation
Distinguishing features	Greasy, flaky eyelid skin (seborrheic blepharitis) Cylindrical collarets, crusty at the eyelashes base (Demodex mites) Hard, fibrinous scales, ring-like formations around the lash shaft (Staphylococcal blepharitis)	Inflammation of the posterior lid margin Meibomian glands appear dilated, obstructed and capped with thickened, waxy, white or yellow secretions Mild pressure to the eyelid expresses abnormal, turbid, or thickened oily secretions Eyelid margin telangiectasias

(continued)

Table 2.1 (continued)

	Anterior blepharitis	Posterior blepharitis
Red flags	Reduced vision Eye pain Intense light sensitivity Unilateral Eyelash loss Not responding to treatment	Reduced vision Severe pain Extreme redness Photophobia Eyelashes loss Trichiasis Changes in eyelids shape Unilateral Not responding to treatment

Eyelid Benign Lesions 3

Eyelid benign lesions (Figs. 3.1, 3.2, 3.3, 3.4, 3.5, and 3.6) can be distinguished from cancerous growths because of their slow growth, well-defined regular borders, symmetry, mobility and lack of bleeding or ulceration.

Different types of benign eyelid lesions have unique identifying features. The following illness scripts (Figs. 3.2, 3.4, and 3.6) and Table 3.1 describe and compare the elements of three common benign lesions (i.e. stye, chalazion and papilloma).

M. Ugarte, *Ophthalmology Illness Scripts*,
https://doi.org/10.1007/978-3-032-31008-8_3

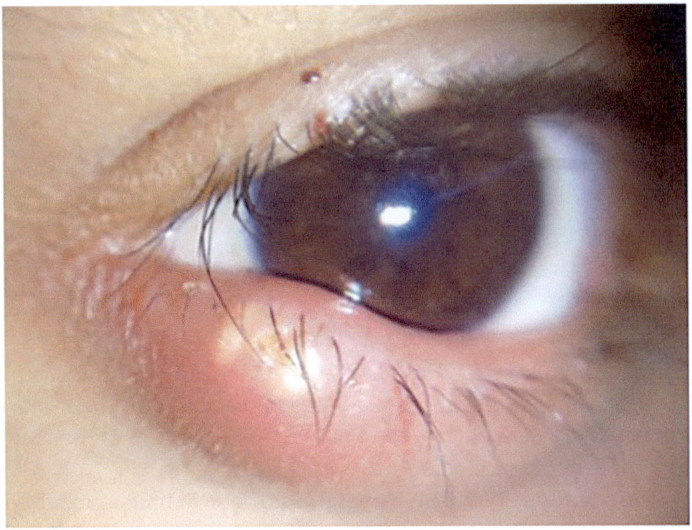

SIGNS

- Red, pus-filled abscess at eyelid margin (external) or deeper within the eyelid (internal)
- Discharge yellow/ white

Fig. 3.1 Stye

CAUSE
- Bacterial infection of eyelid gland or follicle

RISK FACTORS
- Skin conditions (e.g. rosacea)
- Blepharitis
- Poor hygiene
- Eye rubbing
- Systemic conditions (e.g. high cholesterol, diabetes, stress)

MECHANISMS
- Infection
- Inflammation

SYMPTOMS
- Pain
- Crustiness, itchiness, grittiness
- Watery eyes

SIGNS
- Eyelid redness
- Red, pus-filled abscess at eyelid margin (external) or deeper within the eyelid (internal)
- Discharge yellow/ white

POTENTIAL OCULAR COMPLICATIONS
- Abscess growth
- Bleeding
- Persistent pain
- Skin changes, scar
- Eyelid malposition
- Corneal problems
- Extension, periocular, orbital cellulitis
- Loss of vision

NATURAL HISTORY AND PROGNOSIS
- Good prognosis
- Acute
- Most self-limiting within weeks
- Potential recurrences

INVESTIGATIONS
- Biopsy (if persistent, rapidly growing, concerning)

MANAGEMENT
- Lid hygiene
- Pain relief
- Antibiotics eye drops or ointment
- Surgical excision (if causing significant symptoms)

DISTINGUISHING FEATURES
- Red, tenderl lump at the base of an eyelash or gland

RED FLAGS
- Severe or persistent pain
- Pus or blood leaking from the lesion
- Recurrence same location
- No response to treatment
- Extending to the face, cheek
- Reduced vision

Fig. 3.2 Stye illness script (illness script 3)

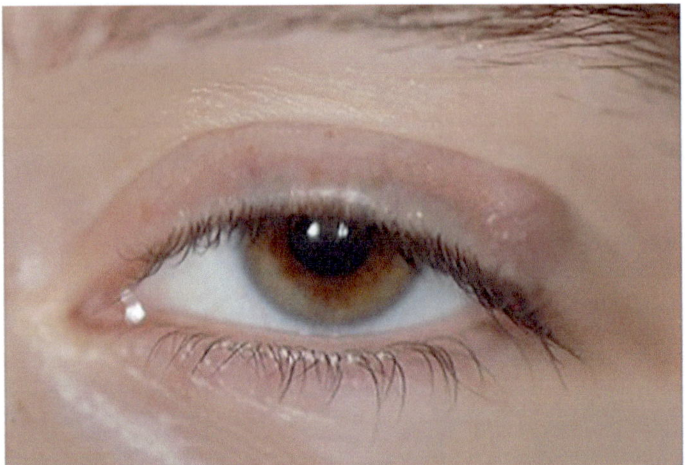

SIGNS

- Nodule within the eyelid (tarsal plate)

Fig. 3.3 Chalazion

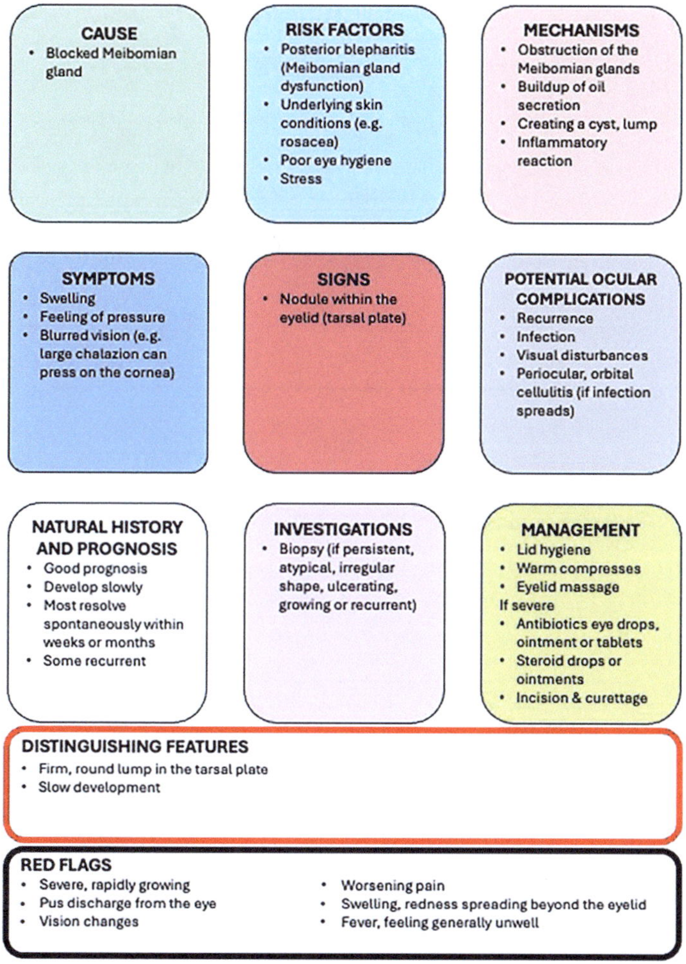

Fig. 3.4 Chalazion illness script (illness script 4)

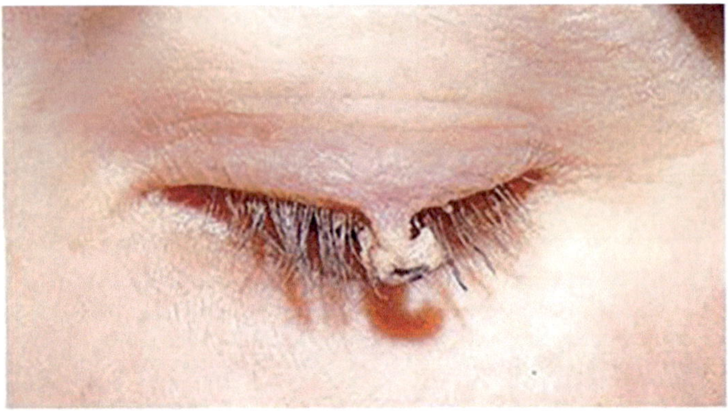

SIGNS

- Soft, flesh-coloured, often pedunculated, growth on eyelid
- Thickened epithelium
- Keratinized surface

Fig. 3.5 Eyelid papilloma

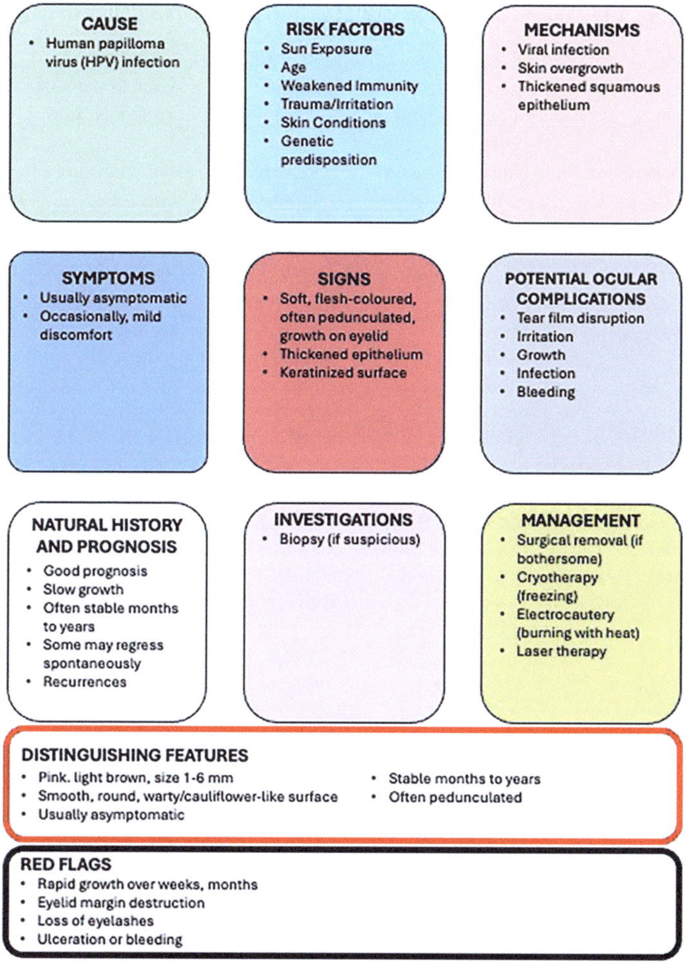

Fig. 3.6 Eyelid papilloma illness script (illness script 5)

Table 3.1 Comparison of stye, chalazion, eyelid papilloma illness scripts

	Stye	Chalazion	Papilloma
Cause	Bacterial infection of eyelid gland or follicle	Blocked Meibomian gland	Human papilloma virus infection
Risk factors	Underlying skin conditions (e.g. rosacea) Blepharitis Poor eye hygiene Eye rubbing Stress Systemic conditions (e.g. elevated cholesterol, diabetes, pregnancy)	Posterior blepharitis (Meibomian gland dysfunction) Underlying skin conditions (e.g. rosacea) Poor eye hygiene Stress	Sun exposure Age Weakened immunity Trauma/irritation Skin conditions Genetic predisposition
Mechanisms and pathogenesis	Bacterial infection of gland or follicle Inflammation	Obstruction of the Meibomian glands Buildup of oil secretion Creating a cyst, lump Inflammatory reaction	Viral infection Skin overgrowth Thickened squamous epithelium
Symptoms	Redness Pain Itchiness Grittiness Crusty eyelids Watery eyes	Pain Feeling of pressure Swelling Blurred vision (e.g. large chalazion can press on the cornea)	Usually asymptomatic Occasionally, mild discomfort
Signs	Red abscess at eyelid margin (external) or deeper within the eyelid (internal) Pus-filled Discharge yellow or white	Nodule within the eyelid (tarsal plate)	Soft, flesh-coloured, often pedunculated, growth Thickened epithelium Keratinized surface

(continued)

Table 3.1 (continued)

	Stye	Chalazion	Papilloma
Complications	Growth Bleeding Persistent pain Chronic skin changes Loss of vision Eyelid thickening and scarring Eyelid malposition Corneal problems Periocular, orbital cellulitis (if infection spreads)	Visual disturbances Recurrence Infection Periocular, orbital cellulitis (if infection spreads)	Tear film disruption Irritation Infection Bleeding Growth
Natural history and prognosis	Acute Most are self-limiting, recover within weeks Some may require medical intervention Recurrences Good prognosis	Develop slowly Most resolve spontaneously within weeks or months Some may require medical intervention Recurrences Good prognosis	Slow growth Often stable for months to years Some may regress spontaneously Recurrences Good prognosis
Investigations	Biopsy for histopathological assessment (if persistent, rapidly growing or concerning)	Biopsy (if persistent, atypical, irregular shape, ulcerating, growing, or recurrent)	Biopsy (if suspicious)

(continued)

Table 3.1 (continued)

	Stye	Chalazion	Papilloma
Management	Hygiene Pain relief Antibiotics eye drops or ointment (for infection) Surgical excision if causing significant symptoms	Hygiene Warm compresses Eyelid massage Antibiotics eye drops or ointment (for infection) Steroid eye drops or ointments (for persistent inflammation) Incision and curettage if problems persist	Surgical removal if bothersome Cryotherapy (freezing) Electrocautery (burning with heat) Laser therapy
Distinguishing features	Tender, red, painful lump At the base of an eyelash	Firm, round lump (within the eyelid tarsal plate) Painless Slow development	Pink, light brown, stable Smooth, round, or rough, warty/cauliflower-like surface, often pedunculated Size is generally small (1–6 mm) Slow growth over months to years Painless and usually asymptomatic No bleeding or discharge

(continued)

Table 3.1 (continued)

	Stye	Chalazion	Papilloma
Red flags	Reduced vision Severe or persistent pain Periocular swelling or redness extending to the face, cheek No response to treatment Pus or blood leaking from the lesion Recurrence in same location	Severe, rapidly worsening pain Swelling, redness spreading beyond the eyelid Vision changes Fever, feeling generally unwell Pus discharge from the eye	Rapid growth over weeks, months Eyelid margin destruction Loss of eyelashes Ulceration or bleeding

4 Eyelid Malposition

Eyelid malposition occurs when an eyelid is not in the correct place against the eyeball (Figs. 4.1, 4.2, 4.3, 4.4, 4.5, and 4.6). In entropion (Fig. 4.1), the eyelid turns inwards. In ectropion (Fig. 4.3), it turns outwards. These conditions usually affect the lower eyelid. Ptosis (Fig. 4.5) is drooping of the upper eyelid. The following entropion, ectropion and ptosis illness scripts (Figs. 4.2, 4.4, and 4.6) and Table 4.1 describe and compare the elements of each condition.

M. Ugarte, *Ophthalmology Illness Scripts*,
https://doi.org/10.1007/978-3-032-31008-8_4

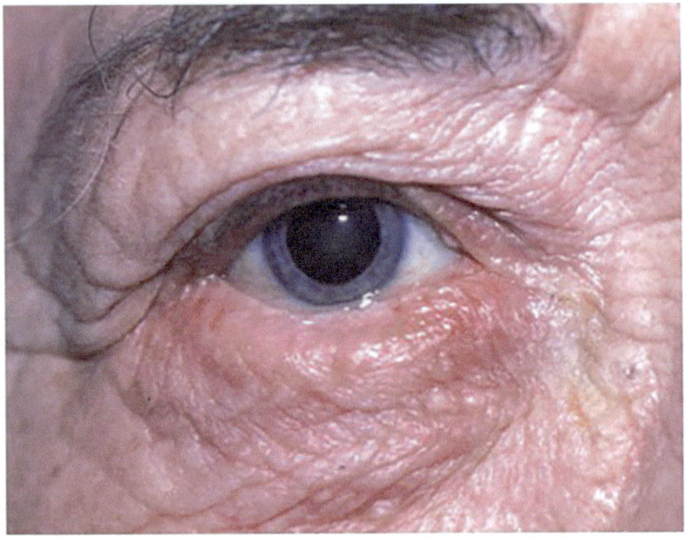

SIGNS

- Eyelid (often lower) margin turn inwards
- Redness
- Inflammation
- Mucous discharge

Fig. 4.1 Entropion

CAUSE
- Muscles weakness
- Muscle spasm
- Conjunctival scarring (cicatricial)
- Mechanical (e.g. swelling, tumours)
- Congenital

RISK FACTORS
- Aging (often > 60 years)
- Chronic inflammation (e.g. blepharitis)
- Skin conditions
- Eyelid laxity (obesity, sleep apnoea)
- Trauma, surgery
- Tumours

MECHANISMS
- Muscle, +/- tendon weakness
- Muscle spasm
- Inflammation
- Scar
- Developmental

SYMPTOMS
- Foreign body sensation
- Eye pain or discomfort
- Watery eyes
- Blurred vision
- Photophobia

SIGNS
- Eyelid (often lower) margin turn inwards
- Redness
- Inflammation
- Mucous discharge
- Eyelid crusting

POTENTIAL OCULAR COMPLICATIONS
- Corneal abrasions
- Corneal ulcers
- Infections
- Corneal scarring
- Permanent vision loss

NATURAL HISTORY AND PROGNOSIS
(depending on cause +/- mechanism)
- Occasional resolution (e.g. mild post-trauma)
- Often progressive
- Good prognosis with early treatment

INVESTIGATIONS
(rarely required)
- Laboratory tests for inflammatory and autoimmune diseases (e.g. ocular pemphigoid, Stevens-Johnson syndrome) (e.g. rare cases of cicatricial entropion)

MANAGEMENT
Temporary measures
- Lubricant eye drops
- Eyelid tape
- Bandage contact lens
- Eyelashes removal
- Botulinum toxin

Surgical correction (if severe, persistent)

DISTINGUISHING FEATURES
- The eyelid turns inward towards the eye
- Commonly affects lower eyelids

RED FLAGS
- Moderate to severe eye pain
- Rapidly increasing red eyes
- Increasing photophobia
- Progressive foreign body sensation
- Decreased vision
- Pus, yellow/green discharge

Fig. 4.2 Entropion illness script (illness script 6)

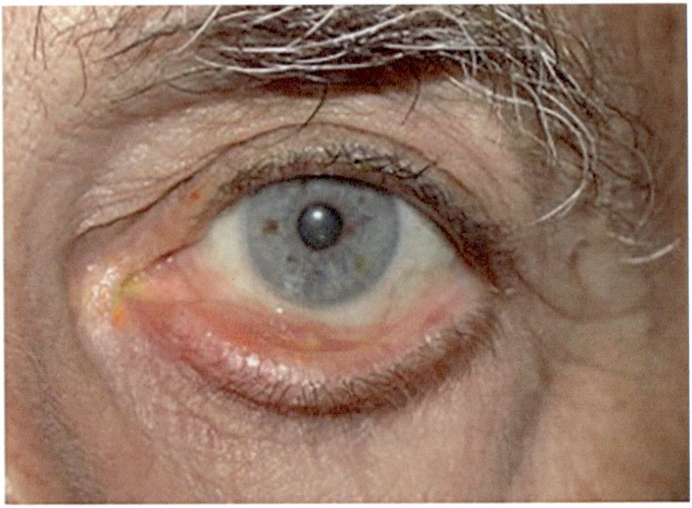

SIGNS

- Droopy/sagging eyelid (usually lower)
- Redness
- Crusting
- Discharge mucous
- Lagophthalmos

Fig. 4.3 Ectropion

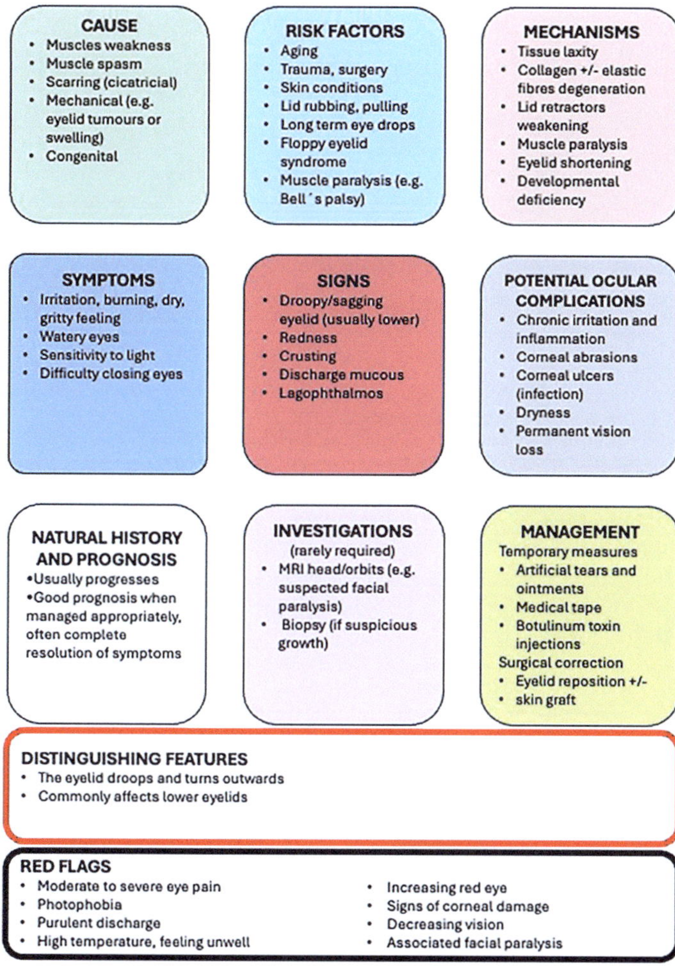

Fig. 4.4 Ectropion illness script (illness script 7)

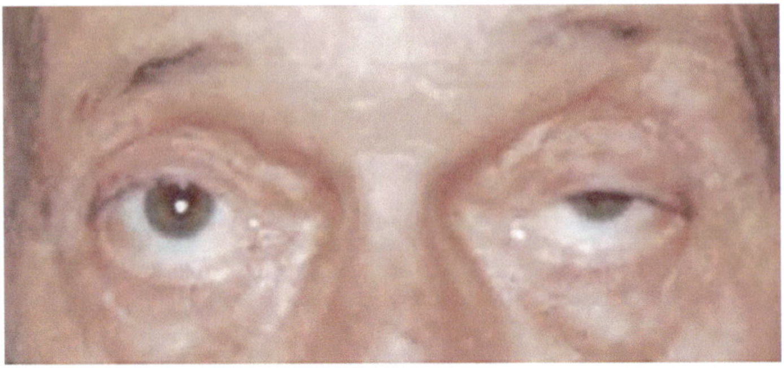

SIGNS

- Drooping of one or both upper eyelids
- Asymmetric appearance
- Compensatory head posturing

Fig. 4.5 Ptosis

CAUSE

- Upper eyelid muscles dysfunction
- Muscle tendon stretch
- Mechanical (e.g. swelling)
- Congenital (e.g. development defect)

RISK FACTORS

- Aging
- Contact lens wear
- Trauma, surgery
- Nerve paralysis (e.g. 3rd CN palsy, Horner's syndrome)
- Muscle diseases (e.g. myasthenia gravis)
- Tumours

MECHANISMS

- Levator muscle aponeurosis stretch +/- disinsertion
- Nerve palsy
- Muscle dysfunction
- Lid movement restriction

SYMPTOMS

- Obstructed visual field
- Impaired vision
- Eye strain and fatigue
- Dry or watery eyes

SIGNS

- Drooping of one or both upper eyelids
- Asymmetric appearance
- Compensatory head posturing

POTENTIAL OCULAR COMPLICATIONS

- Astigmatism
- Amblyopia (children)
- Chronic eye inflammation

NATURAL HISTORY AND PROGNOSIS

- Congenital-typically stable
- Involutional-gradual progression
- Traumatic/inflammatory/neurological may be temporary and resolve with underlying cause

INVESTIGATIONS

(depending on cause +/- presentation)

- Neurological exam
- Muscle function test
- Blood tests (e.g. myasthenia gravis)
- Chest X-rays (e.g. suspected Horner´s syndrome)
- MRI/CT head/orbits

MANAGEMENT

Non-surgical

- Upneeq eye drops (oxymetazoline)
- Ptosis clips fitted to glasses

Surgical

- Levator muscle +/- tendon shortening
- Brow suspension

DISTINGUISHING FEATURES

- Drooping of the upper eyelid

RED FLAGS

- Sudden onset
- Associated pain
- Double vision
- Pupil change

Fig. 4.6 Ptosis illness script (illness script 8)

Table 4.1 Comparison of entropion, ectropion and ptosis illness scripts

	Entropion	Ectropion	Ptosis
Cause	Muscles weakness Muscle spasm Scarring (cicatricial) conjunctiva Mechanical (eyelid tumours or swelling) Congenital conditions	Muscle weakness Muscle spasm Scarring (cicatricial), tightening skin Mechanical, eyelid tumours or swelling Congenital conditions	Reduced function of levator muscle Muscle tendon stretching Mechanical, swelling Muscle weakness/paralysis Congenital causes (e.g. muscle defect)
Risk factors	Ageing (common over 60) Chronic inflammation (e.g. blepharitis) Dry eye syndrome History of trauma, surgery Tumours Infections Skin conditions (e.g. autoimmune) Eyelid laxity (obesity, sleep apnoea)	Ageing Trauma, surgery Skin conditions Eyelid rubbing, pulling Long-term use of eye drops Floppy eyelid syndrome Muscle paralysis (e.g. Bell's palsy)	Ageing Long-term contact lens wear Eye trauma, surgery Nerve paralysis (e.g. stroke, Horner's syndrome, 3rd cranial nerve palsy) Muscle diseases (myasthenia gravis) Tumours

Mechanisms and pathogenesis	Involutional Horizontal lid laxity Weakening of lid support structures Weakening medial and lateral canthal tendons, tarsal plate Lower lid retractor weakness Orbicularis oculi muscle overriding Orbital fat atrophy/ enophthalmos: Cicatricial Scarring contracture of posterior lamella Chronic inflammation Spastic (temporary) Spasm orbicularis oculi muscle Congenital Developmental malformation or dysgenesis of the eyelid structures	Involutional (age-related tissue laxity) Collagen and elastic fibres degeneration in the tarsal plate and canthal tendons Horizontal eyelid lazity Weakening of lid retractors Eversion from the OO contraction Paralytic (OO dysfunction) VII nerve palsy, OO muscle tone loss Cicatricial Shortening eyelid anterior lamella Mechanical Tumour, growth, oedema pull eyelid down and out (gravity and mass effect) Congenital Developmental deficiency or absence of tarsal plate, skin shortage	Aponeurotic Stretching, thinning, or disinsertion of the levator aponeurosis Neurogenic Oculomotor nerve (3rd cranial nerve) palsy: Horner's syndrome Myogenic Dysfunction or disease of lid muscles themselves (myasthenia gravis) Mechanical Excess weight or restricts movement of the eyelid Eyelid tumours (e.g., chalazion), oedema, or scarring, inflammation. Traumatic injury to the eyelid structures Congenital
Symptoms	Foreign body sensation Watery eyes Eye pain or discomfort Photophobia Blurred vision	Watery eyes Dry, gritty feeling Irritation and burning Sensitivity to light and wind Difficulty closing the eye	Obstructed or impaired vision: Eye strain and fatigue Dry or watery eyes

(continued)

Table 4.1 (continued)

	Entropion	Ectropion	Ptosis
Signs	Lower eyelid margin turned inwards Redness and inflammation Mucous discharge Eyelid crusting	Droopy/sagging eyelid Eye and eyelid redness: Discharge mucous Crusting Lagophthalmos	Drooping of one or both upper eyelids Compensatory head posturing Asymmetric appearance
Complications	Corneal abrasions Corneal ulcers Infections Corneal scarring Permanent vision loss	Chronic irritation and inflammation Corneal abrasions Corneal ulcers (infection) Dryness Permanent vision loss	Astigmatism Amblyopia Chronic neck and head problems Psychosocial impact (appearance) Chronic eye inflammation
Natural history and prognosis	Depends on cause and mechanism Occasionally, spontaneous resolution Mild cases (e.g. mild cases post-trauma) Often progressive Good prognosis with early diagnosis and treatment	Usually progresses Prognosis very positive when managed appropriately, symptoms often resolve completely	Congenital typically stable and non-progressive Involutional: gradual progression Traumatic/inflammatory/neurological may be temporary and resolve as the underlying issue heal

Investigations	Laboratory tests for inflammatory and autoimmune diseases, in rare cases of cicatricial entropion with suspected underlying conditions (e.g. ocular pemphigoid, Stevens-Johnson syndrome)	Rarely required MRI head and orbits (in cases with suspected underlying facial paralysis) Biopsy (if suspicious growth)	Depending on the cause and presentation, it might be necessary to carry out: Neurological assessment Muscle function test Blood tests (e.g. myasthenia gravis) Chest X-rays MRI/CT scan head and orbits
Management	Temporary measures Lubricating eye drops Eyelid tape Bandage contact lens Eyelashes removal Botulinum toxin Surgical correction (severe, persistent cases)	Temporary measures Artificial tears and ointments Medical tape Botulinum toxin (Botox) injections Surgical correction Eyelid reposition to its correct place Skin graft (if severe scarring)	Non-Surgical Options Upneeq (oxymetazoline) eye drops temporarily lifts upper eyelid (FDA approved US, not NICE approved UK) Ptosis clips fitted to glasses (physically prop the eyelid up) Surgical treatments Levator muscle or tendon shortening: Brow suspension
Distinguishing features	The eyelid turns inward towards the eye Commonly affects lower eyelids	The eyelid droops and turns outwards Commonly affects lower eyelids	Drooping of the upper eyelid

(continued)

Table 4.1 (continued)

	Entropion	Ectropion	Ptosis
Red flags	Decreased vision Moderate to severe eye pain Progressive foreign body sensation Rapidly increasing red eyes Increasing photophobia Pus-like, sticky, crusty yellow/green discharge	Sudden or decreasing vision Moderate to severe eye pain Increasing red eye Photophobia Headache Signs of corneal damage High temperature, feeling unwell Purulent discharge Associated facial paralysis	Sudden onset Associated pain Double vision Pupil changes

5 Conjunctivitis

Conjunctivitis is inflammation of the conjunctiva, the thin, transparent mucous membrane covering the white part of the eye (sclera) and the inside of the eyelids. It presents with redness (pink) of the white of the eye, gritty, burning or itching sensation, watery or sticky discharge, and crusty eyelids, which can be stuck together, especially in the morning. Potential causes include infections (e.g. bacterial, viral, chlamydial), allergies or irritants (Figs. 5.1, 5.2, 5.3, 5.4, 5.5, 5.6, 5.7, 5.8, 5.9, and 5.10).

The following illness scripts for viral (Fig. 5.2), bacterial (Fig. 5.4), Chlamydial (Fig. 5.6), neonatal (ophthalmia neonatorum) (Fig. 5.8) and allergic conjunctivitis (Fig. 5.10), together with Table 5.1 describe and compare the specific elements for each condition.

M. Ugarte, *Ophthalmology Illness Scripts*,
https://doi.org/10.1007/978-3-032-31008-8_5

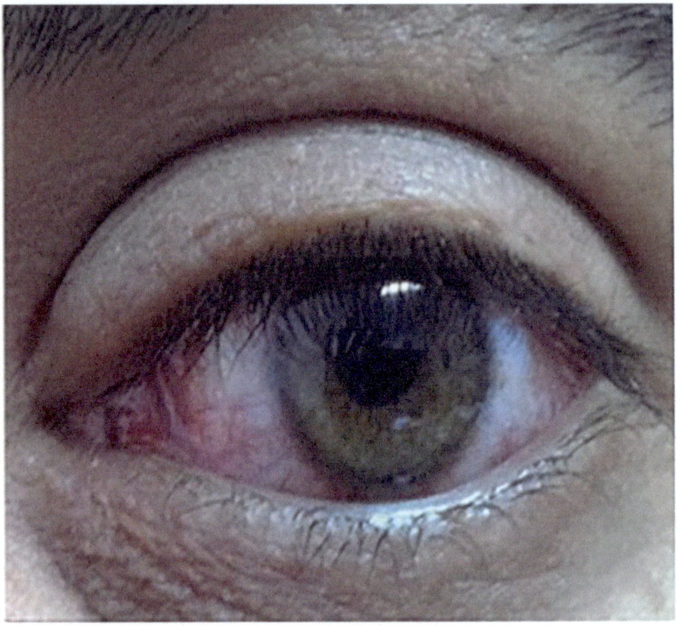

SIGNS

- Red conjunctiva
- Conjunctival follicles
- (Pseudo)membrane
- Discharge watery
- +/-Cornea dryness, stromal infiltrates
- Eyelid swelling
- Preauricular lymphadenopathy

Fig. 5.1 Viral conjunctivitis

CAUSE
Viral infection

Most common
- Adenovirus

Less common
- Coxsackie
- Picornavirus

RISK FACTORS
- URTI
- Contact infected person
- Poor infection control (e.g. hospital stay)

MECHANISMS
- Virus conjunctival colonisation, invasion
- Inflammation
- Immune reaction
- Vasodilation, increase vascular permeability
- Occasional cornea epithelial +/-stromal reaction

SYMPTOMS
- Pain
- Discomfort
- Conjunctival swelling
- +/-Blurred vision
- +/- Photophobia

SIGNS
- Red conjunctiva
- Conjunctival follicles
- (Pseudo)membrane
- Discharge watery
- +/-Cornea dryness, stromal infiltrates
- Eyelid swelling
- Preauricular lymphadenopathy

POTENTIAL OCULAR COMPLICATIONS
- Keratitis
- Corneal scarring

NATURAL HISTORY AND PROGNOSIS
- Usually acute
- Usually self-limiting
- Highly contagious (from one eye to other)

INVESTIGATIONS
- Conjunctival swabs for viral PCR for confirmation (if severe and/or chronic cases)

MANAGEMENT
- Hygiene
- No effective antivirals
- Topical antibiotic (if secondary bacterial infection)
- Topical steroids (e.g. if associated keratitis)

DISTINGUISHING FEATURES
- Discharge watery
- Conjunctival follicles
- Pre-auricular lymphadenopathy
- Sometimes associated keratitis

RED FLAGS
- Severe eye pain
- Marked photophobia
- Eyelid skin rash +/- vesicles
- Severely reduced vision
- White spots on the cornea

Fig. 5.2 Viral conjunctivitis illness script (illness script 9)

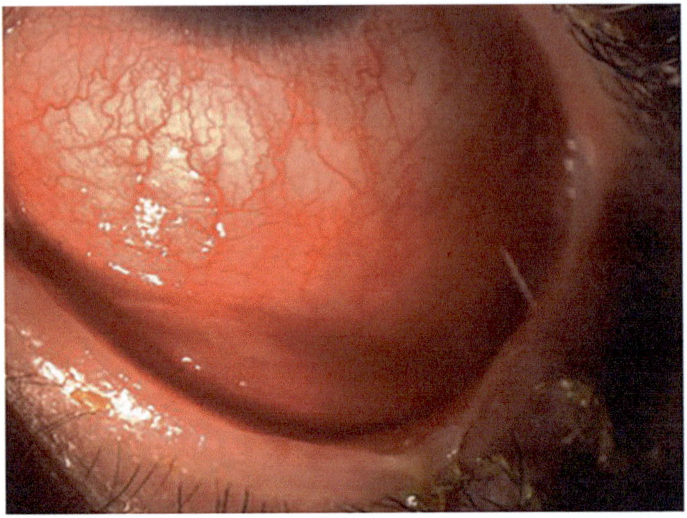

SIGNS

- Red conjunctiva
- Conjunctival papillae
- Membranes or pseudo-membranes
- Discharge sticky, thick, purulent

Fig. 5.3 Bacterial conjunctivitis

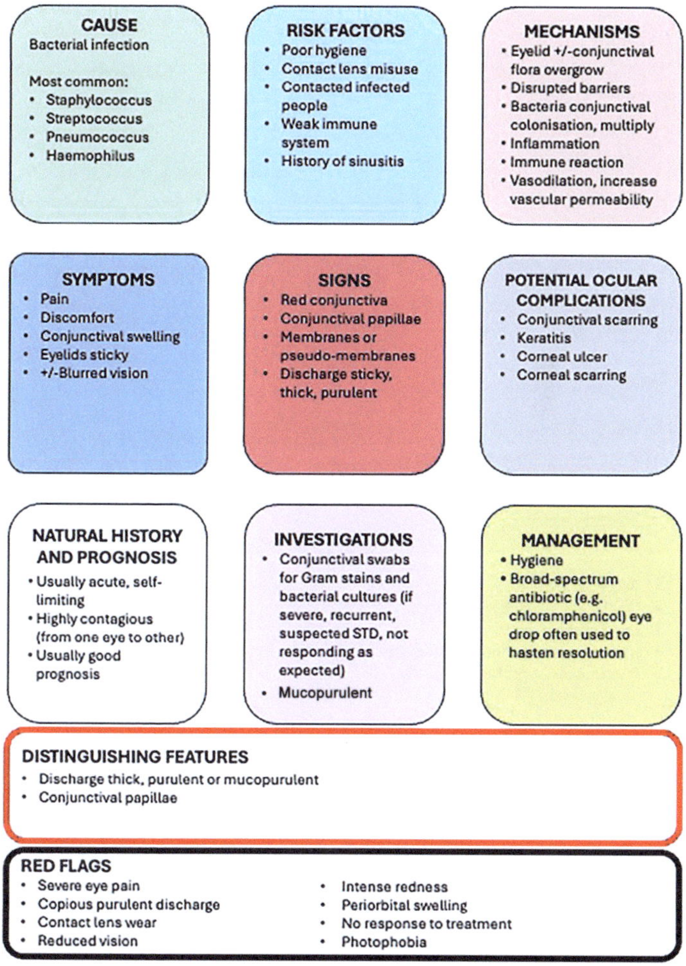

Fig. 5.4 Bacterial conjunctivitis illness script (illness script 10)

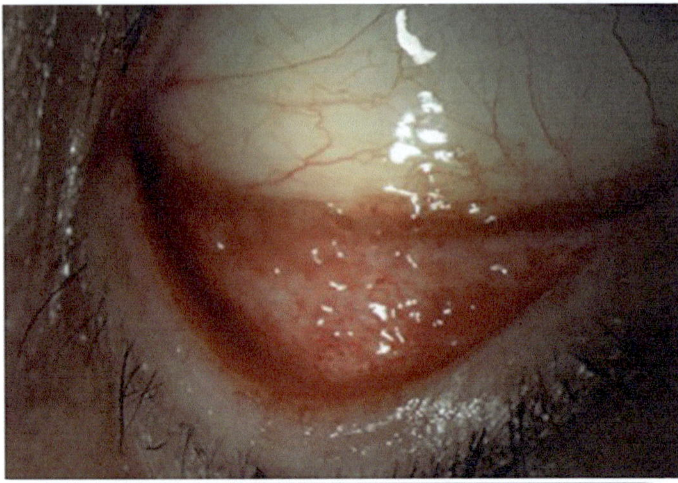

SIGNS

- Red conjunctiva
- Conjunctival follicles
- Discharge mucopurulent
- Cornea micro pannus, subepithelial scarring
- Preauricular lymphadenopathy

Fig. 5.5 Chlamydial conjunctivitis

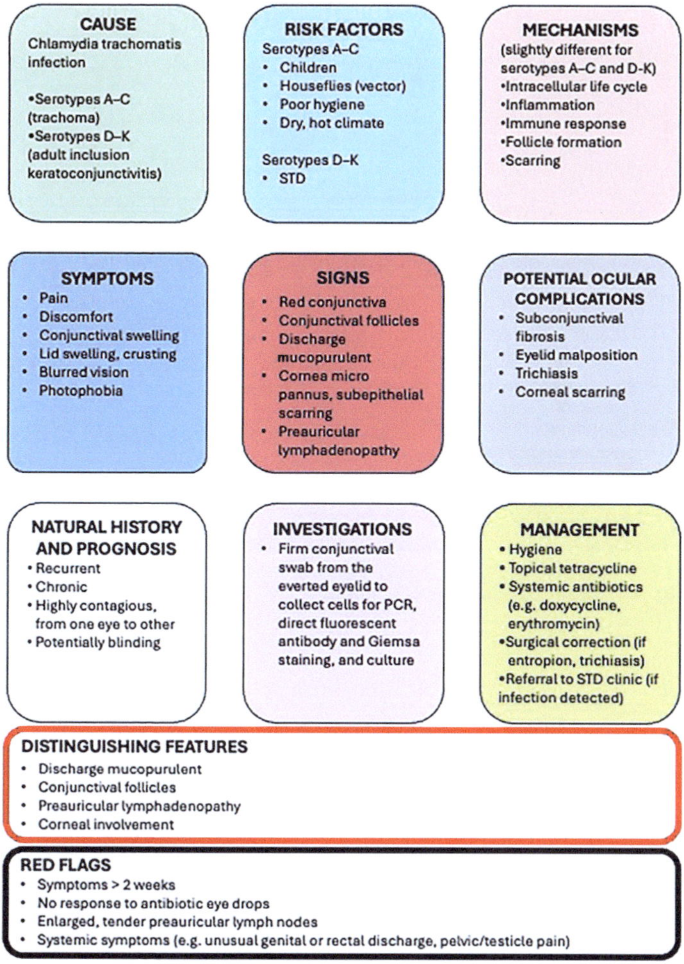

Fig. 5.6 Chlamydial conjunctivitis illness script (illness script 11)

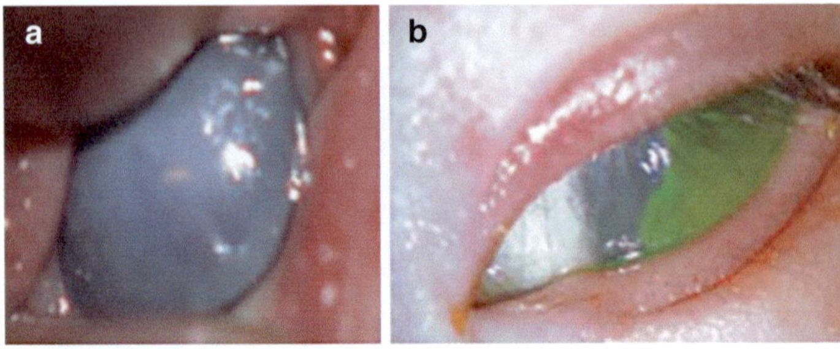

SIGNS
(depending on cause)

- Red conjunctiva
- Follicles
- Membranes
- Eyelid vesicles (HSV)
- Cornea hazy
- Discharge purulent, serosanguinous, mucopurulent

Fig. 5.7 (**a**, **b**) Ophthalmia neonatorum

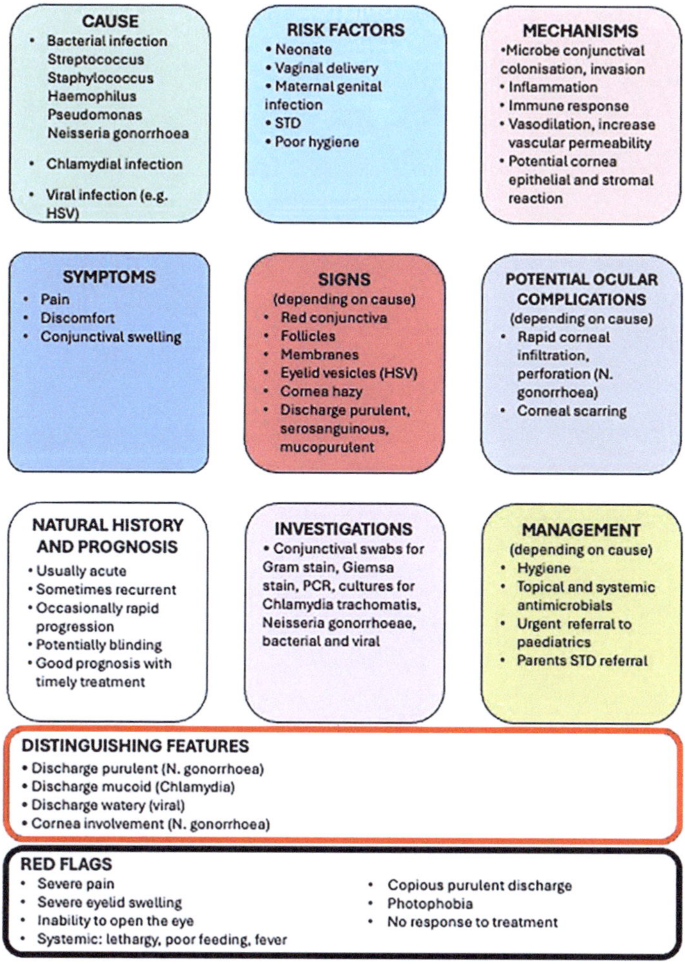

Fig. 5.8 Ophthalmia neonatorum illness script (illness script 12)

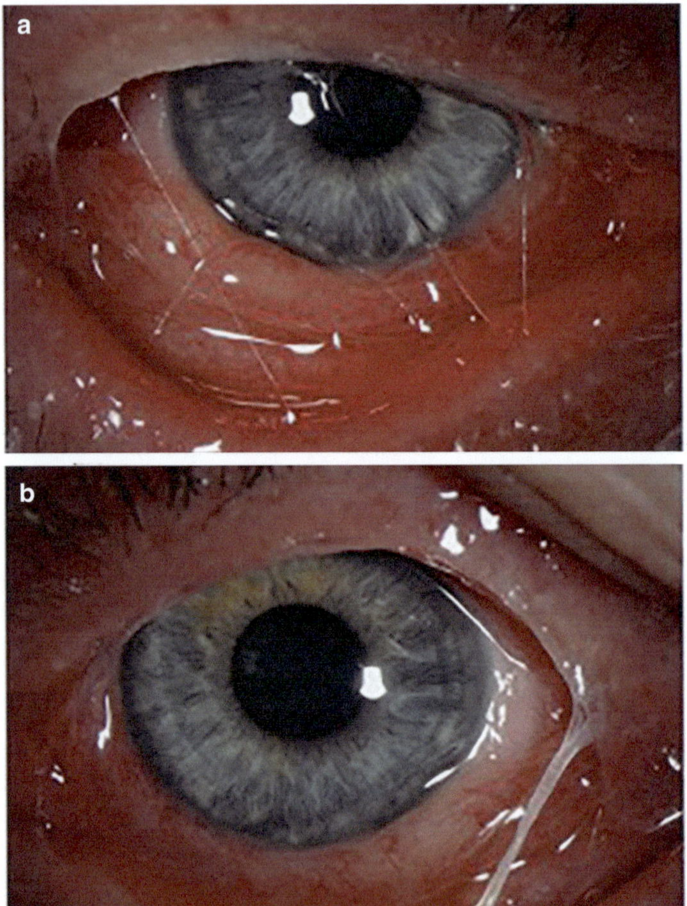

SIGNS

- Conjunctival redness, papillae, swelling (chemosis)
- Discharge watery, mucous, stringy
- Lid oedema
- Corneal punctate epithelial spots +/- shield ulcer

Fig. 5.9 (**a**, **b**) Allergic conjunctivitis

CAUSE
- Airborne allergens (e.g. pollens, ragweed, dust mites)
- Contact lenses, solution
- Eye drops
- Chemicals (e.g. make up)

RISK FACTORS
- Male
- Children
- History of atopy
- Contact lens use
- Eye drops use
- Chemical exposure
- Smoke exposure

MECHANISMS
- Allergen IgE-mediated inflammatory mediators release by mast cells
- Immune cells infiltration
- Vasodilation, increase vascular permeability

SYMPTOMS
- Discomfort
- Conjunctival swelling
- Itchiness
- Photophobia
- Watery, stickiness

SIGNS
- Conjunctival redness, papillae, swelling (chemosis)
- Discharge watery, mucous, stringy
- Lid oedema
- Corneal punctate epithelial spots +/- shield ulcer

POTENTIAL OCULAR COMPLICATIONS
- Subconjunctival fibrosis
- Trichiasis
- Corneal scarring

NATURAL HISTORY AND PROGNOSIS
- Usually acute +/- recurrent (seasonal)
- Occasionally chronic
- Non-contagious
- Good prognosis with timely management

INVESTIGATIONS
- Conjunctival scraping (presence of eosinophils?)
- Allergy testing (if severe, progressive and not responding to treatment)

MANAGEMENT
- Avoid triggering irritant
- Topical mast cell stabilizers
- Topical steroids
- Often necessary to stop contact lens wear

DISTINGUISHING FEATURES
- Intense itching
- Discharge watery, stringy, mucus
- Often bilateral

RED FLAGS
- Severe pain
- Vision changes (blurriness, loss)
- Photophobia
- Contact lens wear

Fig. 5.10 Allergic conjunctivitis illness script (illness script 13)

Table 5.1 Comparison of bacterial, viral, Chlamydial conjunctivitis, ophthalmia neonatorum and allergic conjunctivitis illness scripts

	Bacterial conjunctivitis	Viral conjunctivitis	Chlamydial conjunctivitis	Ophthalmia neonatorum	Allergic conjunctivitis
Cause	Bacterial infection Most common: *Staphylococcus* *Streptococcus* *Pneumococcus* *Haemophilus*	Viral infection Most common Adenovirus Less common Coxsackie Picornavirus	Chlamydial infection *Chlamydia trachomatis* Serotypes A–C (trachoma) Serotypes D–K (adult inclusion keratoconjunctivitis)	Bacterial infection *Streptococcus* *Staphylococcus* *Haemophilus* *Pseudomonas* *Neisseria gonorrhoea* Chlamydial infection Viral infection (e.g. HSV)	Reaction to allergen Airborne allergens Pollens Ragweed Dust mites Contact lenses, solution Eye drops Chemicals (e.g. make up)
Risk factors	Poor hygiene Contact lens misuse Contacted infected people Weak immune system History of sinusitis	URTI Contacted infected person Poor infection control (e.g. hospital stay)	Serotypes A–C Children Houseflies (vector) Poor hygiene Dry, hot climate Serotypes D–K STD	Neonate Vaginal delivery Maternal genital infection STD Poor hygiene	Male Children History of atopy Contact lens use Eye drops use Chemical exposure Smoke exposure

Mechanisms and pathogenesis	Normal flora overgrowth Disrupted natural protective barriers Pathogenic bacteria direct conjunctival epithelium contact Colonize and multiply Inflammation and immune reaction	(Similar to bacteria) Pathogenic viruses direct conjunctival epithelium contact, colonisation, invasion Virus colonisation of cornea epithelium Inflammation Vasodilation	(Similar to bacteria and virus) Serotypes A–C cause trachoma (chronic keratoconjunctivitis) Serotypes D–K cause adult inclusion keratoconjunctivitis	(See bacterial, viral, chlamydial conjunctivitis sections)	Allergen exposure IgE-mediated release of inflammatory mediators (i.e. PG, LT, histamine) by mast cells (type I hypersensitivity) Vasodilation Increased vascular permeability
	Vasodilation Increased vascular permeability	Increased vascular permeability Cornea epithelial and stromal reaction			Immune cells infiltration
Symptoms	Pain Discomfort Conjunctival swelling +/– Blurred vision	Pain Discomfort Conjunctival swelling +/– Blurred vision +/– Photophobia	Pain Discomfort Conjunctival swelling Blurred vision Photophobia	Pain Discomfort Conjunctival swelling	Discomfort Conjunctival swelling Itchiness Photophobia

(continued)

Table 5.1 (continued)

	Bacterial conjunctivitis	Viral conjunctivitis	Chlamydial conjunctivitis	Ophthalmia neonatorum	Allergic conjunctivitis
Signs	Red conjunctiva Conjunctival papillae Membranes or pseudo-membranes Discharge sticky, thick Purulent (pus like) Eyelids stuck together (am) Sinusitis Systemic infection	Red conjunctiva Conjunctival follicles Membranes or pseudo-membrane Discharge watery +/− Cornea SPEEs +/− Cornea stromal infiltrates Eyelid swelling Preauricular lymphadenopathy Cold symptoms Sore throat	Red conjunctiva Conjunctival follicles Discharge Mucopurulent Lid swelling, crusting Cornea micro pannus, subepithelial scarring Preauricular lymphadenopathy Genital infection Urethritis	Red conjunctiva Conjunctival follicles Membranes (*Chlamydia*) Discharge Serosanguinous (Ch) Mucopurulent Purulent-*N. gonorrhoea* Eyelid oedema, vesicles, ulcers (HSV) Cornea hazy Pneumonitis, rhinitis, stomatitis, arthritis, meningitis, septicaemia, CNS signs	Red conjunctiva Conjunctival papillae Swelling (chemosis) Discharge: watery, mucous, stringy Lid oedema Corneal punctate epithelial white spots Shield ulcer Hay fever, runny nose, sneezing, rhinitis
Complications	Keratitis Corneal ulcer Corneal scarring	Keratitis Corneal scarring	Subconjunctival fibrosis Corneal scarring Trichiasis	Rapid corneal infiltration, perforation (*N. gonorrhoea*) Corneal scarring	Subconjunctival fibrosis Corneal scarring Trichiasis

Natural history and prognosis	Acute Usually self-limiting Highly contagious (passed from one eye to the other) Rarely complications	Acute Self-limiting Highly contagious Usually spreads from one eye to the other	Recurrent Chronic Highly contagious, from one eye to fellow eye Potentially blinding	Acute, recurrent Rapid progression Potentially blinding	Acute Chronic Recurrent (seasonal) Non-contagious
Investigations	Conjunctival swabs for Gram stains and bacterial cultures (if severe, recurrent, suspected STD or not responding as expected)	Conjunctival swabs for viral PCR (for confirmation, severe and/or chronic cases)	Firm conjunctival swab from the everted eyelid to collect cells for PCR, direct fluorescent antibody and Giemsa staining, and culture	Conjunctival swabs for Gram stain, Giemsa stain, PCR, cultures for *Chlamydia trachomatis*, *Neisseria gonorrhoeae*, bacterial and viral	Conjunctival scraping Allergy testing (if severe, progressive and not responding to treatment)
Management	Hygiene Broad-spectrum antibiotic (e.g. chloramphenicol) Eye drops often used to hasten resolution	Hygiene No effective commercial antiviral available Topical antibiotic (if secondary bacterial infection)	Hygiene Topical tetracycline Systemic tetracycline: Doxycycline Erythromycin Azithromycin Surgical correction (if entropion and/or trichiasis)	Hygiene (e.g. eye irrigation 0.9% saline) Topical and systemic antimicrobials *Neisseria gonorrhoea* Systemic, 3rd-generation cephalosporin	Avoid triggering irritant Topical mast cell stabilizers Topical steroids Often necessary to stop contact lens wear

(continued)

Table 5.1 (continued)

	Bacterial conjunctivitis	Viral conjunctivitis	Chlamydial conjunctivitis	Ophthalmia neonatorum	Allergic conjunctivitis
		Topical steroids occasionally (e.g. if associated keratitis)	Referral to STD clinic, if infection detected	(ceftriaxone or cefotaxime) im, iv Bacitracin eye ointment *Chlamydia trachomatis* Systemic erythromycin, azithromycin Topical for prophylaxis *Herpes simplex virus* Systemic antiviral Topical antiviral Urgent paediatric opinion Refer parents STD clinic	
Disatinguishing features	Discharge thick, purulent or mucopurulent Conjunctival papillae	Discharge watery Conjunctival follicles Gritty, burning sensation Pre-auricular lymphadenopathy Keratitis	Discharge mucopurulent Conjunctival follicles Preauricular lymphadenopathy Corneal involvement Coexisting genital Chlamydial infection	Discharge purulent (*N. gonorrhoea*) Discharge mucoid (*Chlamydia*) Discharge watery (viral) Cornea involvement (*N. gonorrhoea*)	Discharge watery, stringy, mucus Intense itching FB sensation Often bilateral Severe swollen eyelids Nasal allergy symptoms

Red flags	Severe eye pain Intense redness Reduced vision Photophobia Copious purulent discharge Contact lens wear Periorbital swelling No response to treatment Systemic illness	Severe eye pain Severely reduced vision Marked photophobia Pupil changes White spots on the cornea Systemic: fever, lethargy, confusion, skin rash Contact lens wear	Symptoms >2 weeks No response to antibiotic eye drops Enlarged, tender preauricular lymph nodes Systemic symptoms (e.g. unusual genital or rectal discharge, pelvic/testicle pain)	Severe pain Copious purulent discharge Severe eyelid swelling Photophobia Inability to open the eye Herpes infection signs No response to treatment Systemic: lethargy, poor feeding, fever	Severe pain Vision changes (blurriness, loss) Photophobia Small pupil Thick yellow/green discharge Eye crusting Contact lens wear

6 Keratitis

Keratitis is inflammation of the cornea, the transparent dome-shape tissue at the front of the eye. Common symptoms and signs are eye pain, gritty and foreign body sensation, as well as excessive tearing, redness, blurred vision, photophobia and sometimes a hazy or opaque cornea (Figs. 6.1, 6.2, 6.3, 6.4, 6.5, 6.6, 6.7, and 6.8). Infectious keratitis can be caused by bacteria, viruses, fungi and parasites. Non-infectious keratitis can be caused by a relatively minor injury, such as from wearing contact lenses for long periods of time or foreign body in the eye. Interstitial keratitis is inflammation of the corneal stroma often from infections (e.g. syphilis, viruses) or autoimmune condition. It is an immune-mediated response, not usually a direct surface infection, leading to scarring and new blood vessel growth in the cornea. It requires prompt treatment (if early diagnosis) with corticosteroids and managing the underlying cause to prevent scarring and permanent vision loss.

The following illness scripts (Figs. 6.2, 6.4, 6.6, and 6.8) and Table 6.1 describe and compare the elements of each condition. Key distinguishing features involving both specific symptoms and clinical signs (i.e. appearance of the corneal infiltrate) help identify the underlying cause (viral, bacterial, fungal, protozoan-Acanthamoebal, autoimmune).

M. Ugarte, *Ophthalmology Illness Scripts*,
https://doi.org/10.1007/978-3-032-31008-8_6

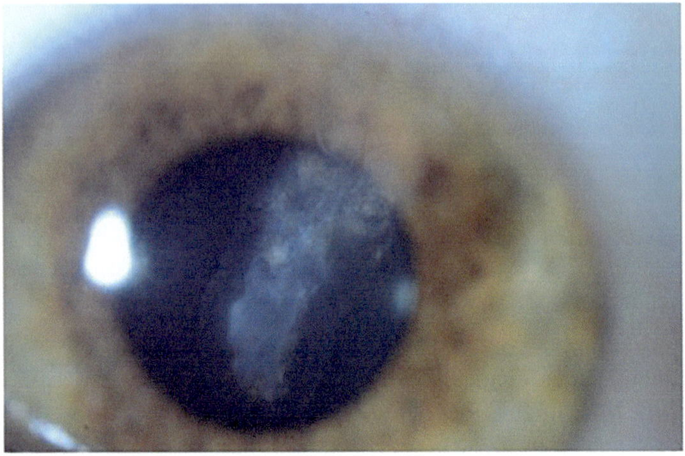

SIGNS

Cornea:

- Dendritic ulcer (fluorescein dye)
- Haze, oedema
- Stromal opacity
- +/-Neovascularisation
- +/-Iritis
- +/-Eyelid blisters

Fig. 6.1 Viral keratitis

CAUSE

Viral infection

Most common:
- Herpes simplex virus 1 (HSV1)
- Varicella zoster virus (VZV)

RISK FACTORS
- Dry eye
- Trauma, surgery
- Poor lid closure
- Contact lens wear
- Long-term steroid drops
- History of cold sores
- Herpes zoster ophthalmicus

MECHANISMS
- Virus corneal epithelium invasion
- Inflammation
- Hyper-sensitivity to viral antigens
- Corneal stromal oedema, reduced sensation, ulceration

SYMPTOMS
- Redness, ciliary injection
- Mild-moderate discomfort, pain
- Discharge watery
- Reduced corneal sensation
- Visual loss
- Photophobia

SIGNS

Cornea:
- Dendritic ulcer (fluorescein dye)
- Haze, oedema
- Stromal opacity
- Neovascularisation

Potentially associated:
- Iritis
- Eyelid blisters

POTENTIAL OCULAR COMPLICATIONS
- Corneal scarring, neovascularisation, perforation
- Secondary glaucoma

NATURAL HISTORY AND PROGNOSIS
- Acute
- Recurrent (e.g. immunosuppress)
- Occasionally chronic
- Potentially blinding

INVESTIGATIONS
- Corneal scrapes or swabs for PCR and culture

MANAGEMENT
- Antivirals (e.g. aciclovir) topical, oral
- Antibiotics topical (prevent 2nd infection)
- Steroids topical with caution (if stromal involvement)
- Corneal graft (if severe scarring)

DISTINGUISHING FEATURES
- Corneal ulcer appearance (fluorescein dye drops staining): dendritic, geographic
- Reduced corneal sensation
- Recurrence
- Discharge clear, watery

RED FLAGS
- Severe pain
- Photophobia
- Thick yellow/green discharge
- Vision changes (blurriness, loss)
- Small pupil
- Contact lens wear

Fig. 6.2 Viral keratitis illness script (illness script 14)

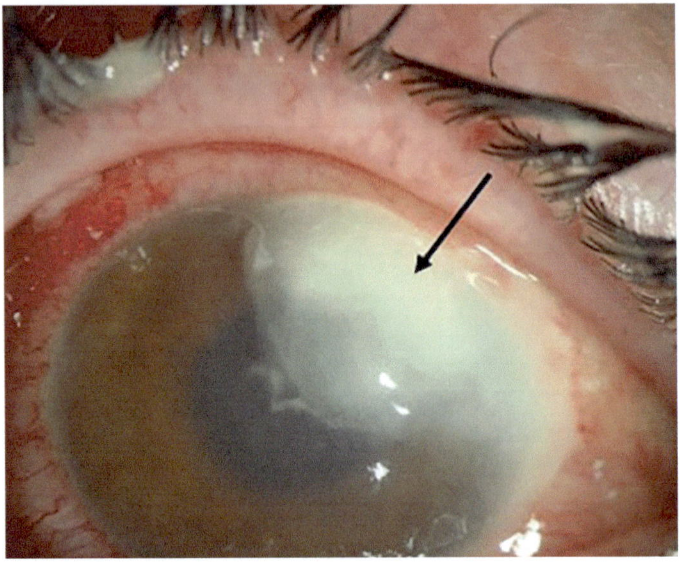

SIGNS

- Corneal surface defect (ulcer)
- White/gray spot
- Conjunctival injection, chemosis
- +/- associated iritis
- +/- hypopyon
- +/- purulent discharge

Fig. 6.3 Bacterial keratitis

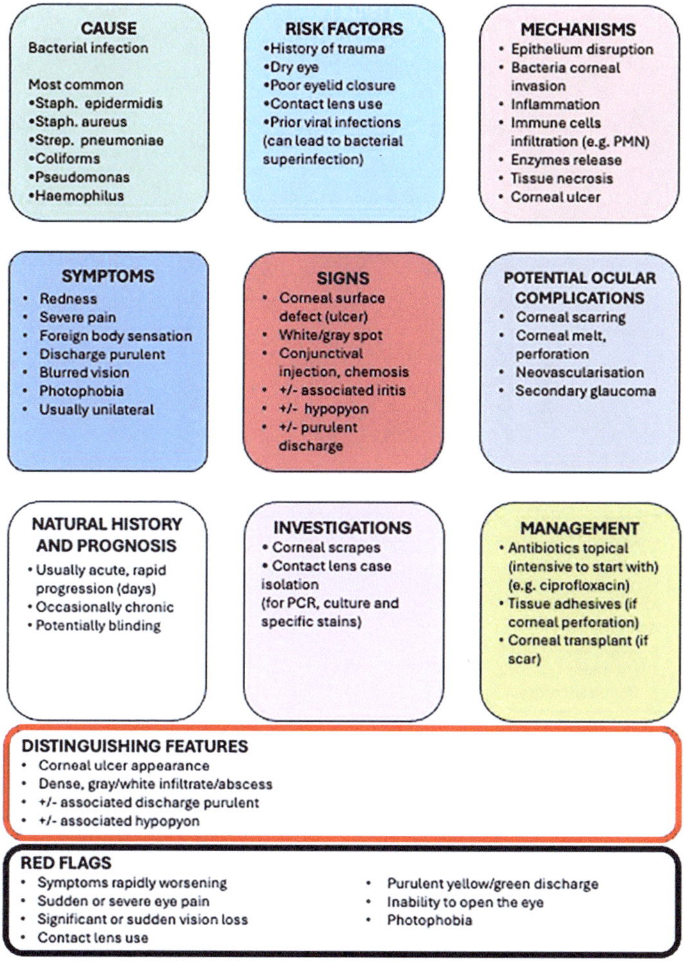

Fig. 6.4 Bacterial keratitis illness script (illness script 15)

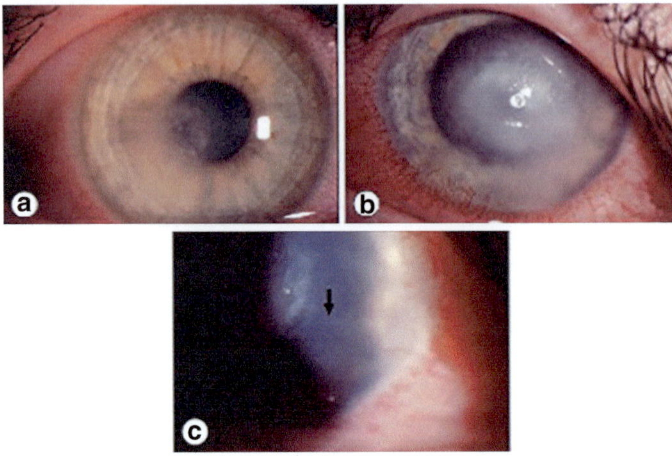

SIGNS

Fungus

- Atypical infiltrates
- Satellite lesions
- +/- iritis
- +/- hypopyon

Acanthamoeba

- Atypical infiltrates
- Prominent nerves
- Pseudodentrites
- +/-scleritis

Fig. 6.5 **a**, **b** and **c** Fungal or Acanthamoebal keratitis

CAUSE
- Fungal infection
or
- Acanthamoebal infection

RISK FACTORS
- Warmer climates
- Trauma with vegetable matter (fungus)
- Contact lens use
- Swimming with contact lenses on
- Long term use topical antibiotics and/or steroids

MECHANISMS
Fungus:
- Stromal invasion, infiltrate, replication
- Inflammation
- Tissue necrosis
- Satellite lesions

Acanthamoeba:
- Epitheliopathy
- Radial keratopathy
- Perineural infiltrates

SYMPTOMS
- Redness
- Extremely painful (Acanthamoeba)
- Discharge purulent
- Blurred vision
- Photophobia
- Usually unilateral

SIGNS
Fungus
- Atypical infiltrates
- Satellite lesions
- +/- iritis
- +/- hypopyon

Acanthamoeba
- Atypical infiltrates
- Prominent nerves
- Pseudodentrites
- +/-scleritis

POTENTIAL OCULAR COMPLICATIONS
- Corneal scarring
- Perforation
- Neovascularisation
- Secondary glaucoma

NATURAL HISTORY AND PROGNOSIS
- Chronic
- Slower onset (weeks)
- Potentially blinding

INVESTIGATIONS
- In vivo confocal microscopy (direct visualization)
- Corneal scrapes, swabs (for special stains, PCR, cultures)

MANAGEMENT
Fungus:
- Antifungals topical (e.g. natamycin, voriconazole, amphotericin)

Acanthamoeba:
- Topical chlorhexidine, PHMB, propamidine (treatment for months)

DISTINGUISHING FEATURES
- Chronic symptoms, unresponsive to standard antibiotic
- Severe disproportionate pain (*Acanthamoeba*)
- Corneal atypical infiltrates: *Fungus*: multiple surrounding smaller "satellite" lesions; *Acanthamoeba:* radial perineural

RED FLAGS
- Rapid worsening of symptoms
- Sudden or significant vision loss
- Severe pain
- Poor treatment response

Fig. 6.6 Fungal or Acanthamoebal keratitis illness script (illness script 16)

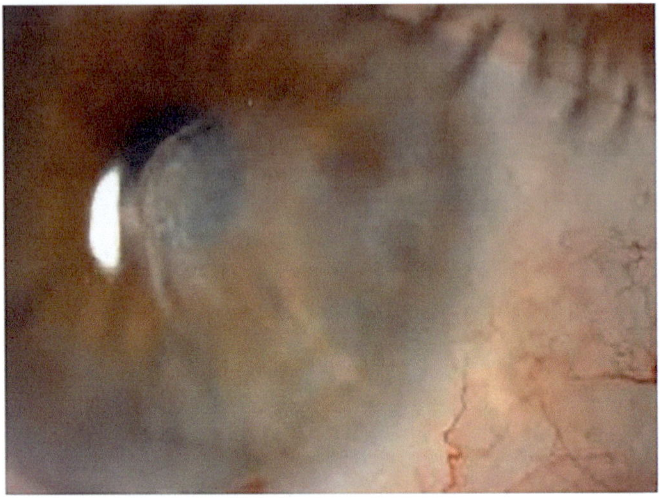

SIGNS

- No corneal epithelial fluorescein dye stain
- Stromal haze, diffuse opacification
- Mid stroma scar
- Stroma empty ('ghost') blood vessels, neovascularization

Fig. 6.7 Interstitial keratitis

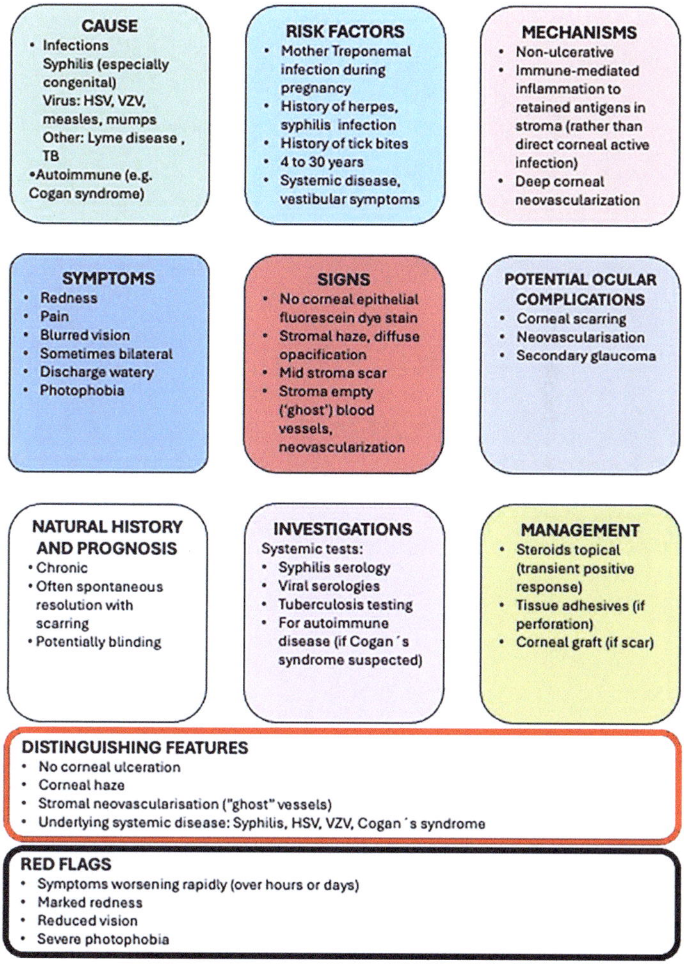

Fig. 6.8 Interstitial keratitis illness script (illness script 17)

Table 6.1 Comparison of viral, bacterial, fungal, Acanthamoebal and interstitial keratitis illness scripts

	Viral keratitis	Bacterial keratitis	Fungal or Acanthamoeba keratitis	Interstitial keratitis
Cause	Viral infection Most common: Herpes simplex virus 1 (HSV1) Varicella zoster virus (VZV)	Bacterial infection Most common (normal lid flora) *Staphylococcus epidermidis* *Staphylococcus aureus* *Streptococcus pneumoniae* *Coliforms* *Pseudomonas* *Haemophilus*	Fungal infection Acanthamoebal infection	Infections Syphilis (especially congenital) Virus: HSV, VZV, measles, mumps Other: Lyme disease Autoimmune (e.g. Cogan syndrome)
Risk factors	Dry eye History of surgery, trauma Inadequate eyelid closure Contact lens wear Prolonged use topical steroids History of cold sores, HZO, varicella	History of trauma Dry eye Inadequate eyelid closure Contact lens use Prior viral infections (can lead to bacterial superinfection)	Warmer climates Trauma with vegetable matter (fungus) Contact lens use Swimming with contact lenses Long-term use topical antibiotics and/or steroids	Systemic disease, vestibular symptoms Mother Treponemal infection during pregnancy History of herpes infections, tick bites, syphilis 4–30 year-old range

Mechanisms and pathogenesis	Direct viral infection of corneal epithelial cells Immune hypersensitivity to viral antigens Inflammation Corneal stromal oedema Corneal scarring Damage to the corneal nerves Reduced corneal sensation Impaired healing Corneal ulceration	Epithelium disruption Microbial invasion of stroma Inflammation Immune cells infiltration (e.g. PMN) Enzymes release (e.g. proteases) Tissue necrosis Corneal ulcer Corneal scarring Corneal melt, perforation	*Fungus*: Stromal invasion, infiltrate and replication Inflammation Tissue necrosis Satellite lesions *Acanthamoeba*: Epitheliopathy Radial keratopathy Perineural infiltrates	Non-ulcerative Immune-mediated inflammation to retained antigens in stroma (rather than direct, active infection of corneal cells) Deep corneal neovascularization
Symptoms	Redness, ciliary injection Pain (mild-moderate discomfort) Visual loss Discharge watery, tearing Reduced corneal sensation Photophobia Systemically unwell, lid (HZO)	Redness Severe pain FB sensation Blurred vision Discharge purulent Photophobia	Redness Extremely painful (*Acanthamoeba*) Discharge purulent Blurred vision Photophobia	Redness Pain Blurred vision Bilateral Lacrimation: Photophobia

(continued)

Table 6.1 (continued)

	Viral keratitis	Bacterial keratitis	Fungal or Acanthamoeba keratitis	Interstitial keratitis
Signs	Dendritic ulcers (HSV, VZV) Punctate epithelial erosions Epithelial oedema focal, diffuse Superficial corneal haze Stromal oedema Increased corneal thickness White stromal opacity Endotheliitis Keratic precipitates Cornea neovascularization Associated iritis, eyelid blisters, vesicles, distribution V1 (HZO)	Corneal surface defect (ulcer) Focal white/grey corneal spot (well-defined borders) Conjunctival injection Conjunctival chemosis +/– Associated iritis +/– Associated hypopyon +/– Associated purulent discharge	*Fungus* Atypical corneal infiltrates: Feathery/serrated margins Raised surface and edges Satellite lesions Often associated with iritis Hypopyon *Acanthamoeba* Corneal infiltrate feathery border Prominent, infiltrated, corneal nerves, pseudodentrites Associated scleritis (advanced)	No epithelial involvement Stromal haze, diffuse opacification Mid stromal scar Stromal neovascularization, empty (“ghost”) blood vessels
Complications	Corneal scarring Perforation Secondary glaucoma Neovascularization	Corneal scarring Perforation Secondary glaucoma Neovascularization	Corneal scarring Perforation Secondary glaucoma Neovascularization	Corneal scarring Secondary glaucoma Neovascularization

Natural history and prognoss	Acute Recurrence (e.g. immunosuppression) Chronic Potentially blinding	Acute rapid progression (days) Chronic Potentially blinding	Chronic slower onset (weeks) Potentially blinding	Chronic Often spontaneous resolution with scarring Potentially blinding
Investigations	Corneal scrapes or swabs for PCR and culture	Corneal scrape Contact lens case isolation For PCR, culture and specific stains	In vivo confocal microscopy for direct visualization Corneal scrapes, swabs for PCR, culture and special stains	Systemic tests: may involve syphilis serology, viral serologies and tuberculosis testing
Management	Topical antivirals (e.g. aciclovir, ganciclovir) Oral antiviral (e.g. aciclovir) Topical antibacterials (prevent secondary infection) Topical steroids (if stromal involvement, cautiously; not in dendritic ulcer, may exacerbate) Corneal graft (if severe scarring)	Topical antibiotics (intensive to start with) Dual therapy to cover most organisms (e.g. cefuroxime and gentamicin) Monotherapy (e.g. ciprofloxacin) Tissue adhesives (if corneal perforation) (cyanoacrylate glue) Corneal transplant	*Fungus:* Topical antifungals Natamycin Voriconazole Amphotericin *Acanthamoeba:* Topical chlorhexidine Poly hexamethylene biguanide (PHMB) Propamidine Treatment for months often	Topical steroids (transient positive response to steroids support the diagnosis) Tissue adhesives (if perforation) Corneal graft (if corneal scarring)

(continued)

Table 6.1 (continued)

	Viral keratitis	Bacterial keratitis	Fungal or Acanthamoeba keratitis	Interstitial keratitis
Distinguishing features	Corneal ulcer appearance (fluorescein staining) Dendritic Geographic Reduced corneal sensation Discharge clear, watery History of HSV or VZV infection Recurrence	Corneal ulcer appearance Well-defined borders Dense, grey/white, yellow/white infiltrate/abscess +/– Associated discharge purulent +/– Associated hypopyon	Chronic symptoms Unresponsive to standard antibiotic Corneal appearance: *Fungal*: Dry, raised, firm surface Infiltrates feathery, irregular margins, multiple surrounding smaller "satellite" lesions *Acanthamoeba* Punctate epitheliopathy or pseudodendrites (early phase) Ring-shaped, radial perineural (advanced) Transparent, dot-like, multifocal Severe disproportionate pain	Corneal haze No corneal ulceration Stromal neovascularization Significant pain Photophobia Underlying systemic disease: Syphilis, HSV, VZV Cogan's syndrome (immune-mediated systemic vasculitis)

Red flags	Reduced vision Moderate to severe pain Photophobia White/grey cornea Branching dendritic ulcer on the cornea Reduced corneal sensation Blisters, rash eyelid or forehead	Symptoms rapidly worsening Sudden or severe eye pain Significant or sudden vision loss White/grey spot on the cornea Photophobia Purulent yellow/green discharge Inability to open the eye History of contact lens wear Recent eye trauma or surgery	Rapid worsening of symptoms Sudden or significant vision loss Severe pain White/grey spot on the cornea Poor treatment response	Symptoms worsening rapidly (over hours or days) Moderate to severe eye pain Reduced vision Marked redness Severe photophobia Excessive tearing or discharge Corneal haze or opacity

Uveitis

7

Uveitis is an inflammation of the uvea (the middle layer of the eye), including the iris (the visible coloured part), ciliary body and choroid. It is primarily distinguished by: (a) anatomical location (anterior, intermediate, posterior, panuveitis), (b) nature of the onset, duration and course (acute, chronic, recurrent), (c) laterality (unilateral, bilateral, alternating), (d) association with specific symptoms, signs and underlying conditions (HLAB27, juvenile idiopathic arthritis, sarcoid) and e) pathology (granulomatous, non-granulomatous) (Figs. 7.1, 7.2, 7.3, 7.4, 7.5, and 7.6).

Anterior uveitis (i.e. iritis) is the result of inflammation in the iris and/or ciliary body (Figs. 7.1 and 7.2). Intermediate uveitis is inflammation in the vitreous and peripheral retina (Figs. 7.3 and 7.4). Posterior uveitis is the inflammation of the retina and/or choroid (Figs. 7.5 and 7.6).

Uveitis can be caused by infections (HSV, VZV, CMV, *Toxoplasma gondii*, syphilis, tuberculosis), inflammatory conditions (e.g. associated with HLAB27, sarcoid, Behcet's disease) or be of unknown origin (idiopathic). Certain conditions can mimic uveitis (masquerades syndromes), such as intraocular lymphoma.

Common symptoms include eye pain, redness, photophobia and visual symptoms (e.g. blurred, cloudy vision, sometimes floaters and flashing lights). Ocular signs (some require slit lamp examination) include white or yellow deposits on the corneal

M. Ugarte, *Ophthalmology Illness Scripts*,
https://doi.org/10.1007/978-3-032-31008-8_7

endothelium (keratic precipitates), white blood cells and proteins (flare) in the anterior chamber, adhesions of the iris to the lens (posterior synechiae) causing pupil distortion sometimes small and irregular.

The illness scripts for anterior uveitis (Fig. 7.2), intermediate uveitis (Fig. 7.4), posterior uveitis (Fig. 7.6) and Table 7.1 describe and compare the elements of each type of uveitis. Key distin-

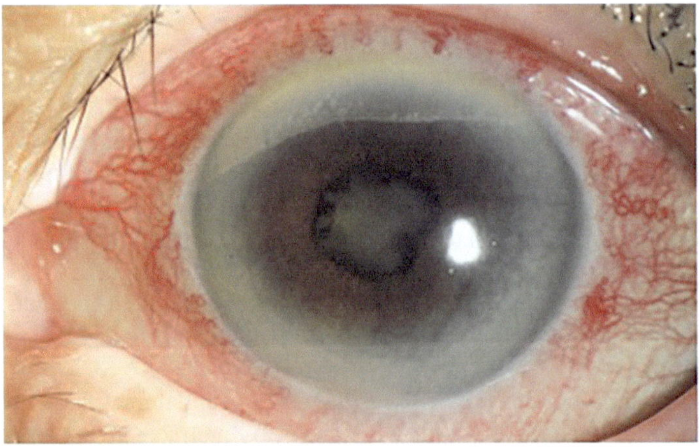

Fig. 7.1 anterior uveitis

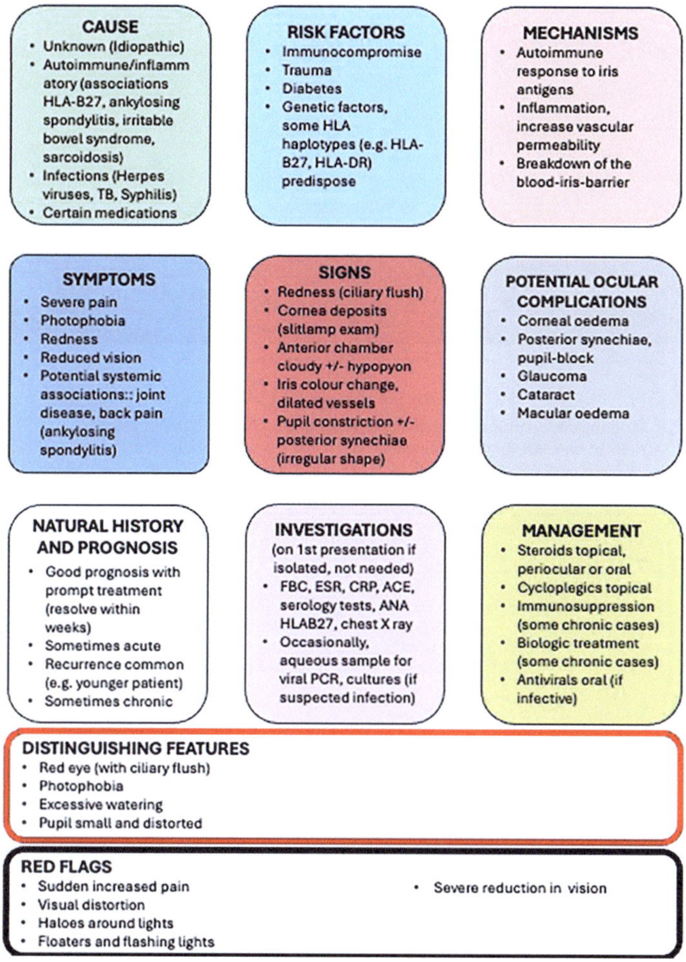

Fig. 7.2 Anterior uveitis illness script (illness script 18)

guishing features involving both specific symptoms and clinical signs and red flags are highlighted.

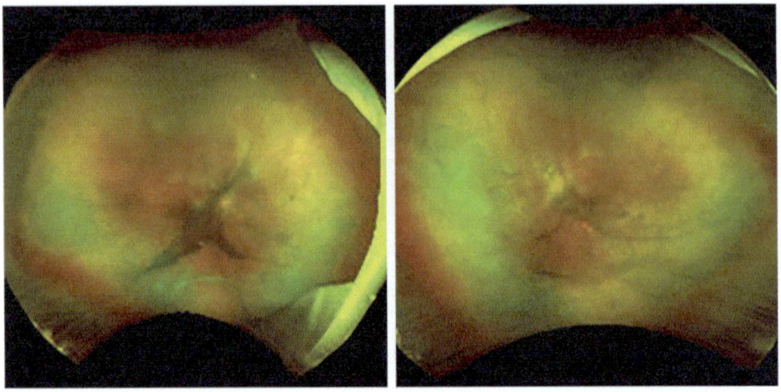

SIGNS

- Vitreous cells, inflammatory material and proteins (vitritis) (slitlamp exam)
- Retina vasculitis (peripheral retina)
- Macular oedema

Fig. 7.3 Intermediate uveitis

CAUSE
- Unknown (idiopathic)
- Autoimmune(inflammatory (e.g. associated MS, sarcoid)
- Infective (e.g. TB, syphilis, Lyme disease)

RISK FACTORS
- Immunocompromise
- Diabetes
- Autoimmune conditions: MS, sarcoid, Infection (e.g. TB)
- Genetic factors

MECHANISMS
- Inflammation, autoimmune
- Immune cells infiltration
- BRB breakdown
- Macrophages stimulation
- T cells activation
- Cytokines release
- Tissue damage

SYMPTOMS
- Floaters
- Blurred vision
- Visual distortion
- Not much pain
- Some photophobia
- Some redness
- Potential systemic associations

SIGNS
- Vitreous cells, inflammatory material and proteins (vitritis) (slitlamp exam)
- Retina vasculitis (peripheral retina)
- Macular oedema

POTENTIAL OCULAR COMPLICATIONS
- Cataract
- Glaucoma
- Macular oedema
- Epiretinal membrane
- Retinal detachment
- Optic disc swelling

NATURAL HISTORY AND PROGNOSIS
- Chronic
- Generally good long-term visual prognosis with adequate management

INVESTIGATIONS
(based on presentation)
- Optical coherence tomography
- Fundus angiography
- Chest X ray
- MRI head
- Aqueous, vitreous (for PCR, cultures)
- Ocular ultrasound

MANAGEMENT
(sometimes long term)
- Steroids topical, periocular, intraocular, oral
- Systemic immuno-suppression (some cases)
- Monoclonal antibodies (some cases)

DISTINGUISHING FEATURES
- Floaters
- Blurred vision
- Vitreous haze, cells, aggregates of cells
- Inflammation of retinal vessels

RED FLAGS
- Severe eye pain, headache
- Significant reduction in vision
- Photophobia
- Pupil irregularities

Fig. 7.4 Intermediate uveitis illness script (illness script 19)

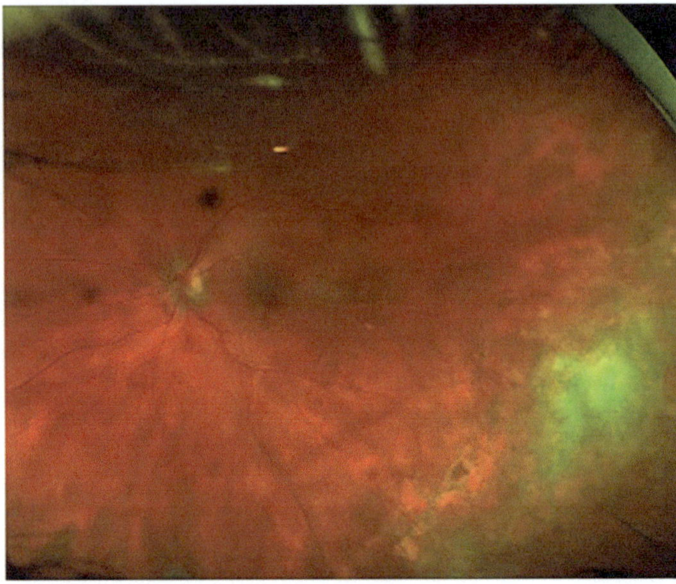

SIGNS:

- Vitritis, vitreous haze (proteins and cells)
- Retina vasculitis
- Retinitis
- Choroidal lesions
- Chorioretinal scars
- +/-choroidal and retina neovascularisation
- +/- macular oedema
- +/- swollen optic disc

Fig. 7.5 Posterior uveitis

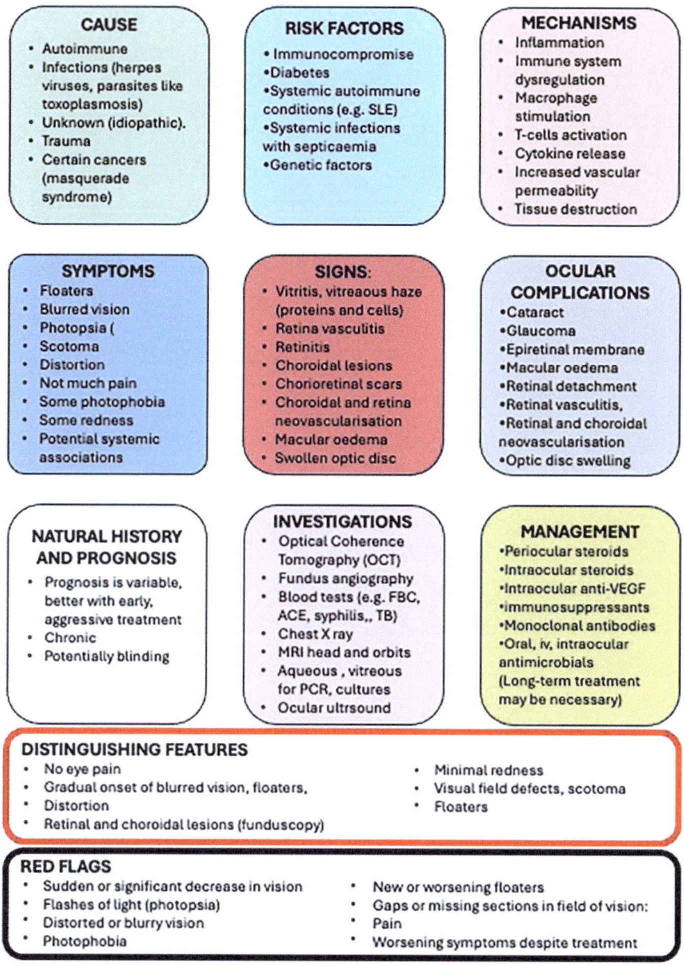

Fig. 7.6 Posterior uveitis illness script (illness script 20)

Table 7.1 Comparison of anterior, intermediate and posterior uveitis illness scripts

	Anterior uveitis	Intermediate uveitis	Posterior uveitis
Cause	Unknown (idiopathic) Autoimmune/inflammatory (associated with ankylosing spondylitis, irritable bowel syndrome, sarcoidosis, HLA-B27) Infections (herpes viruses, TB, syphilis) Certain medications	Unknown (idiopathic) Autoimmune (inflammatory (associated with MS, sarcoid) Infective (TB, syphilis, Lyme disease)	Autoimmune (associated with rheumatoid arthritis, sarcoidosis) Infections (herpes viruses, parasites like toxoplasmosis) Unknown (idiopathic) Trauma Certain cancers (masquerade syndrome)
Risk factors	Immunocompromise Trauma Diabetes Genetic factors, some HLA haplotypes (e.g., HLA-B27, HLA-DR), predispose	Immunocompromise Diabetes Systemic autoimmune conditions: MS, sarcoid, infection (e.g. tuberculosis) Genetic factors	Immunocompromise Diabetes Systemic autoimmune conditions (e.g. SLE) Systemic infections with septicaemia Genetic factors

Mechanisms and pathogenesis	Autoimmune response to iris antigens (presumed molecular mimicry, proteins of an infective agent) Inflammation Increased vascular permeability Breakdown of the blood-iris-barrier Adjacent structures may be involved	Inflammation Autoimmune response to eye antigens (molecular mimicry by infective agent) Increased vascular permeability Breakdown of the BRB Immune cells infiltration Stimulation of macrophages Activation of T cells Cytokines release Swelling and tissue damage	Inflammation Immune system dysregulation Macrophage stimulation T cells (e.g. autoreactive Th17) infiltration and activation Cytokine release Increased vascular permeability Tissue destruction

(continued)

Table 7.1 (continued)

	Anterior uveitis	Intermediate uveitis	Posterior uveitis
Symptoms	Severe pain Redness Photophobia Reduced vision Potential systemic associations: joint disease Back pain (ankylosing spondylitis) Juvenile idiopathic arthritis (e.g. children) Reiter disease	Floaters Blurred vision Visual distortion Not much pain Some photophobia Some redness Potential systemic associations Respiratory symptoms (e.g. sarcoid, TB) Joint disease Skin problems Bowel disease: ulcerative colitis, Crohn disease and Whipple disease Infectious: syphilis, herpetic disease (HSV, VZV), CMV Neurological symptoms: MS	Floaters Blurred vision Photopsia (flashes of light) Scotoma Distortion Not much pain Some photophobia Some redness Potential systemic associations Respiratory symptoms (sarcoidosis or TB) Joint disease Skin problems: sarcoid, Behçet disease, psoriasis Bowel disease: ulcerative colitis, Crohn disease and Whipple disease Infections: syphilis, herpetic disease (HSV, VZV), CMV.

Signs	Redness (with ciliary flush) Pupil constriction (miosis) Iris changes in colour and texture Posterior synechiae (irregular pupil) from adhesions of iris to lens capsule Slit lamp exam, aqueous humour in anterior chamber cloudy (white cells, proteins), fibrin, hypopyon Inflammatory cells on corneal endothelium (keratic precipitates) Iris nodules, dilated blood vessels	Slit lamp examination and fundoscopy: Vitreous cells and proteins (haze) (vitritis) Snowballs Snowbanking (deposits of inflammatory material at the pars plana and ora serrata) Retina vasculitis (peripheral retina) Macular oedema	Slit lamp examination and fundoscopy: Vitritis, vitreaous haze (proteins and cells) Retina vasculitis Retinal whitening, infiltrate, retinitis Choroidal lesions Chorioretinal scars Choroidal and retina neovascularization Macular oedema Swollen optic disc

(continued)

Table 7.1 (continued)

	Anterior uveitis	Intermediate uveitis	Posterior uveitis
Complications	Corneal oedema Cataract Posterior synechiae, pupil-block Glaucoma Macular oedema	Cataract Glaucoma Macular oedema Epiretinal membrane Retinal detachment Optic disc swelling	Cataract Glaucoma Epiretinal membrane Macular oedema Retinal detachment Retinal vasculitis, vascular occlusions Retinal and choroidal neovascularization Optic disc swelling
Natural history and prognosis	Usually good prognosis with prompt treatment (resolving within weeks) Recurrence common (e.g. younger patients) Occasionally chronic	Generally good long-term visual prognosis Chronic condition	Prognosis is variable Chronic Prognosis better with early, aggressive treatment Potentially blinding

Investigations	First presentation does not need investigations unless systemic symptoms FBC, ESR, CRP, ACE, serology tests, ANA HLAB27, chest X ray Occasionally aqueous sample for viral PCR and cultures (if suspected viral infection)	Optical coherence tomography Fluorescein angiography Indocyanine green angiography Chest X ray MRI head (if suspected CNS pathology) Aqueous and vitreous samples for PCR, cultures (if suspected infection) Ocular ultrasound (if no fundal view)	Optical coherence tomography Fluorescein angiography Indocyanine green angiography Blood tests (e.g. FBC, ACE, syphilis, Lyme serology, TB test) Chest X ray MRI head and orbits Aqueous and vitreous samples for PCR, cultures (in suspected infections) Ocular ultrasound (if no fundal view. If suspected posterior scleritis)
Management	Topical steroids Topical cycloplegics (e.g. cyclopentolate) Periocular injection of steroids (e.g. subconjunctival, orbital floor, sub-Tenon space) Intraocular injection of steroids ORAL steroids Systemic immunosuppression Monoclonal antibodies (e.g. Adalimumab) Oral antiviral if infection Long-term treatment may be necessary	Topical steroids Periocular injection of steroids (e.g. subconjunctival, orbital floor, sub-Tenon space) Intraocular injection of steroids Oral steroids Systemic immunosuppressants: antimetabolites (e.g. azathioprine, methotrexate and mycophenolate), calcineurin inhibitors (e.g. cyclosporine), alkylating agents (e.g. cyclophosphamide) Monoclonal antibodies Long-term treatment may be necessary	Steroids injected onto the orbital floor or into the sub-Tenon space Intraocular steroids Intraocular anti-VEGF (if intraocular neovascularization) Systemic immunosuppressants: antimetabolites (e.g. azathioprine, methotrexate and mycophenolate), calcineurin inhibitors (e.g. cyclosporine), alkylating agents (e.g. cyclophosphamide) Monoclonal antibodies Oral, iv, intraocular antimicrobials Long-term treatment may be necessary

(continued)

Table 7.1 (continued)

	Anterior uveitis	Intermediate uveitis	Posterior uveitis
Distinguishing features	Painful Red eye (with ciliary flush) Photophobia Excessive watering Blurred vision Pupil small and distorted	Minimal eye pain Minimal readmes Blurred vision Floaters Vitreous haze, cells, aggregates of cells Inflammation and sheathing of peripheral retinal vessels Minimal anterior chamber reaction	No eye pain Minimal redness Gradual onset of blurred vision, floaters Visual field defects, scotoma Distortion Floaters Retinal and choroidal lesions (funduscopy)
Red flags	Sudden pain Red eye Photophobia Blurred vision Dull ache worse with focus Watery eyes Floaters Small/irregular pupil	Severe eye pain Significant reduction in visual acuity worsening symptoms despite treatment Photophobia Pupil irregularities New-onset headache, nausea, vomiting neurological symptoms	Sudden or significant decrease in vision New or worsening floaters Flashes of light (photopsia) Gaps or missing sections in field of vision: Distorted or blurry vision: Pain Photophobia Worsening symptoms despite treatment

8 Episcleritis and Scleritis

Episcleritis is generally a benign, self-limiting condition characterized by inflammation of the episclera, the clear tissue between the sclera (the white outer layer of the eye) and the conjunctiva (Figs. 8.1 and 8.2). It causes mild superficial redness (sector or diffuse), mild discomfort and tearing, often in one eye, with no vision loss, light sensitivity or significant discharge.

Scleritis, inflammation of the sclera (the white outer layer of the eye), on the other hand, is a very serious condition, with potential irreversible vision loss (Figs. 8.3 and 8.4). It is frequently associated with an underlying autoimmune condition (e.g. rheumatoid arthritis). Occasionally, it can be associated with an infection. Its symptoms include severe, dull, aching pain (worse on eye movements, which can wake patient from sleep at night) and intense redness in the deeper vessels with a blue-red hue (not blanching with phenylephrine eye drops). Depending on the location and type, scleritis can be classified into anterior or posterior; nodular, diffuse, necrotizing or non-necrotizing. Anterior scleritis is the most common (90% of all cases). It presents with visible redness at the front. Posterior scleritis affects the back of the eye. It may have normal front appearance. On B-ultrasound scan, it shows thickened posterior sclera and optic nerve. Necrotizing scleritis can result in severe tissue melting.

M. Ugarte, *Ophthalmology Illness Scripts*,
https://doi.org/10.1007/978-3-032-31008-8_8

In this chapter, we present the illness scripts for episcleritis (Fig. 8.2) and scleritis (Fig. 8.4). In Table 8.1, we describe and compare the elements of each condition. Key distinguishing features and red flags are highlighted.

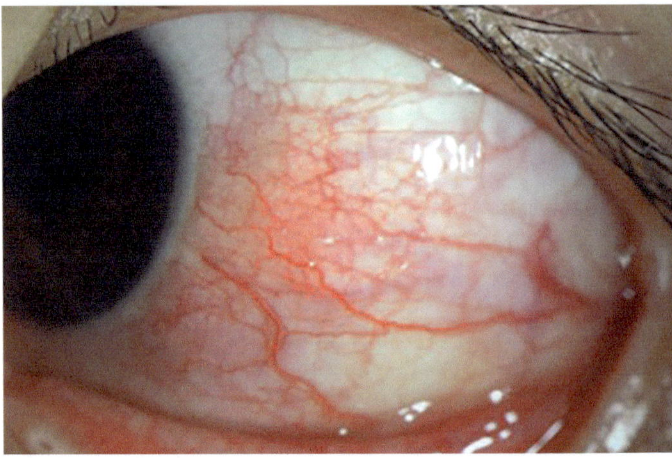

SIGNS:

- Bright red area on the eye surface
- Sectorial or diffuse
- Redness bleaches (turns white) with 2.5% phenylephrine eye drops

Fig. 8.1 Episcleritis

CAUSE
- Idiopathic (unknown)
- Dry eye
- Rarely autoimmune (15-30% associated systemic condition)

RISK FACTORS
- Rarely associated with systemic disease (e.g. Sjogren´s syndrome, connective tissue disorders)

MECHANISMS
- Episcleral blood vessels inflammation

SYMPTOMS
- Sudden onset
- Redness
- Mild discomfort, grittiness, foreign body sensation

SIGNS:
- Bright red area eye surface
- Sectorial or diffuse
- Redness bleaches (turns white) with 2.5% phenylephrine eye drops

POTENTIAL OCULAR COMPLICATIONS
- Insignificant

NATURAL HISTORY AND PROGNOSIS
- Usually acute, self-limiting, resolution (1-2 weeks)
- Some recurrences
- Rarely chronic
- Benign, excellent prognosis

INVESTIGATIONS
- Blood tests for underlying systemic connective tissue disorders (in unresolving, chronic cases)

MANAGEMENT
- Lubricant eye drops
- Anti-inflammatories topical (if significant discomfort)
- Nonsteroidal anti-inflammatories orally (in very rare, severe disease)

DISTINGUISHING FEATURES
- Superficial diffuse patch or nodular redness (movable)
- Redness blanches with phenylephrine 2.5% eye drops
- Mild pain or tenderness
- Majority no systemic association

RED FLAGS
- New or worsening symptoms
- Photophobia
- History of autoimmune or inflammatory diseases

Fig. 8.2 Episcleritis illness script (illness script 21)

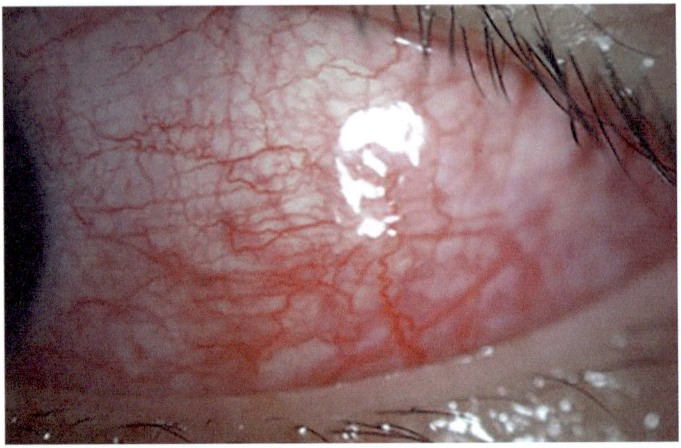

SIGNS

- Deep diffuse or nodular redness (blue, purple, no blanching with phenylephrine drops)
- +/- necrosis and uveal exposure
- Posterior scleritis (no redness sometimes)

Fig. 8.3 Scleritis

CAUSE
- Unknown (idiopathic)
- Autoimmune (>50% systemic association)
- Infections (bacterial, viral or fungal)

RISK FACTORS
- Collagen disease
- Vascular disease
- Rheumatoid arthritis
- Granulomatous polyangiitis
- Polyarteritis nodosa
- Systemic lupus erythematosus

MECHANISMS
- Inflammation
- Immune complex dependent microangiopathy
- Ischaemia
- Necrosis

SYMPTOMS
- Deep, severe pain (worse at night, with eye movement))
- Blurred vision
- Photophobia
- Discharge watery
- Potential systemic associations

SIGNS
- Deep diffuse or nodular redness (blue, purple, no blanching with phenylephrine drops)
- Occasional, necrosis and uveal exposure
- Posterior scleritis (no redness sometimes)

POTENTIAL OCULAR COMPLICATIONS
- Scleral thinning, perforation
- Peripheral keratitis
- Uveitis
- Cataract
- Glaucoma
- Choroidal effusions (posterior scleritis)

NATURAL HISTORY AND PROGNOSIS
- Gradual onset
- High risk of relapse
- Potentially blinding
- Permanent visual loss if not treated promptly

INVESTIGATIONS
- Chest X ray
- Blood tests (for potential systemic associations)
- Ultrasound B scan (assessment of posterior scleritis)

MANAGEMENT
- Non-steroidal anti-inflammatories oral
- Steroids topical, oral or intravenous
- Immunosuppressants
- Monoclonal antibodies
- Scleral grafting (if risk of scleral perforation)

DISTINGUISHING FEATURES
- A violaceous, non-blanching redness, red-blue hue
- Deep, boring, radiating pain, worsens with eye movement and at night
- Often (50%) association with autoimmune or inflammatory diseases

RED FLAGS
- Increased pain
- Progressive reduction in vision
- Scleral thinning, revealing underlying choroid (bluish area)
- Swollen optic disc and/or retinal detachment

Fig. 8.4 Scleritis illness script (illness script 22)

Table 8.1 Comparison of episcleritis and scleritis illness scripts

	Episcleritis	Scleritis
Cause	Idiopathic (unknown) Dry eye Rarely autoimmune (15–30% associated systemic condition)	Unknown (idiopathic) Autoimmune (>50% associated with autoimmune conditions Infections: bacterial, viral or fungal
Risk factors	Rarely associated with systemic disease (e.g. Sjogren's syndrome, connective tissue disorders)	Collagen disease Vascular disease Rheumatoid arthritis Granulomatous polyangiitis Polyarteritis nodosa Systemic lupus erythematosus
Mechanisms and pathogenesis	Episcleral blood vessels inflammation	Inflammation Immune complex dependent microangiopathy Ischaemia Necrosis
Symptoms	Sudden onset Redness Mild discomfort Grittiness Foreign body sensation Normal vision	Deep, severe eye pain that may radiate to the jaw, forehead, ear, often worse at night and with eye movement Intense redness with a bluish or purplish hue Tenderness to touch Photophobia Blurred vision Discharge watery Potential associations: rheumatoid arthritis, SLE, gout, etc.
Signs	Bright red area of the eye Sectorial or diffuse Redness bleaches (turn white) with 2.5% phenylephrine drops	Deep red, bluish-purple hue, does not blanch with phenylephrine drops Diffuse or nodular scleral swelling Occasionally necrosis, uveal exposure Anterior sclera might not look red in posterior scleritis

(continued)

Table 8.1 (continued)

	Episcleritis	Scleritis
Complications	Insignificant	Scleral thinning, perforation (scleromalacia perforans) Peripheral keratitis (sometimes ulcerative) Uveitis Cataract Glaucoma Choroidal effusions (posterior scleritis)
Natural history and prognosis	Usually self-limiting Acute, rapid resolution usually within 1–2 weeks Rarely chronic	Potentially blinding Permanent visual loss if associated complications
Investigations	Blood tests for underlying systemic connective tissue disorders (in unresolving, chronic cases)	Chest X-ray Blood tests Ultrasound B scan (assessment of posterior scleritis)
Management	Topical lubricants Topical anti-inflammatories (if significant discomfort) Systemic nonsteroidal anti-inflammatories (in rare, severe disease)	Topical steroids Systemic anti-inflammatories (non-steroidal, steroids, immunosuppressants) Monoclonal antibodies (e.g. adalimumab) and tumour necrosis factor (alpha inhibitors (e.g. infliximab) (refractory non-infectious cases) Scleral grafting (if risk of scleral perforation)
Distinguishing features	Superficial redness diffuse patch or nodular (movable) Redness blanches with phenylephrine drops Mild pain or tenderness Normal vision Majority no systemic association	A violaceous, non-blanching redness, red-blue hue Deep, boring, radiating pain, worsens with eye movement and at night Potential vision loss (especially posterior uveitis) Often (50%) association with autoimmune or inflammatory diseases

(continued)

Table 8.1 (continued)

	Episcleritis	Scleritis
Red flags	New or worsening symptoms Photophobia History of autoimmune or inflammatory diseases	Increased pain Progressive reduction in vision Scleral thinning, revealing underlying choroid (bluish area) Severe photophobia Excessive watering Lid swelling, proptosis, swollen optic disc and/or retinal detachment (signs of posterior scleritis)

9 Cataracts

A cataract is the natural ageing process of the crystalline lens with protein breakdown resulting in gradual, painless lens clouding leading to various visual symptoms (e.g. blurred vision, glare, faded colours, difficulty with night vision) that gradually worsen over time.

Cataracts are classified by where they form in the lens (Figs. 9.1, 9.2, 9.3, 9.4, 9.5, and 9.6). The three main types are nucleosclerotic (yellowing of the centre of lens) (Figs. 9.1 and 9.2), cortical (spoke-like opacities in the cortex of the lens) (Figs. 9.3 and 9.4) and posterior subcapsular (at the back of lens, which can cause fast-progressing glare symptoms) (Figs. 9.5 and 9.6). Other types of cataract include congenital, traumatic and secondary (e.g. in cases of intraocular inflammation).

The following illness scripts (Figs. 9.2, 9.4, and 9.6) and Table 9.1 describe and compare the elements of nucleosclerotic, cortical and posterior subcapsular cataracts.

M. Ugarte, *Ophthalmology Illness Scripts*,
https://doi.org/10.1007/978-3-032-31008-8_9

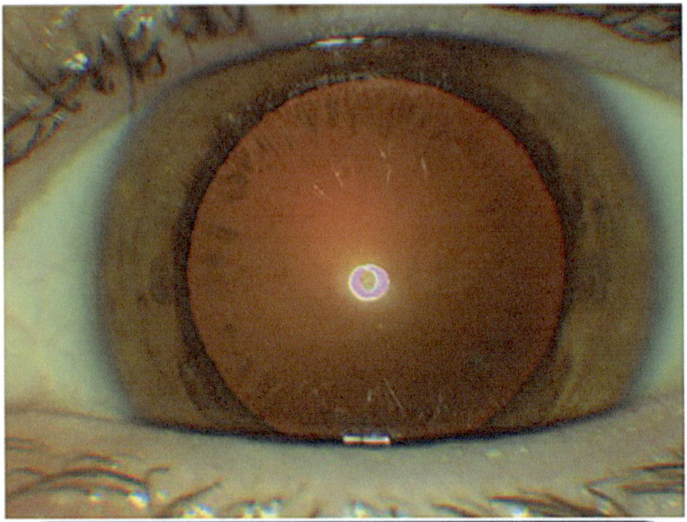

SIGNS

- Dull red reflex
- Lens centre appearance: yellow/brown
- "Oil-drop"

Fig. 9.1 Nucleosclerotic cataract

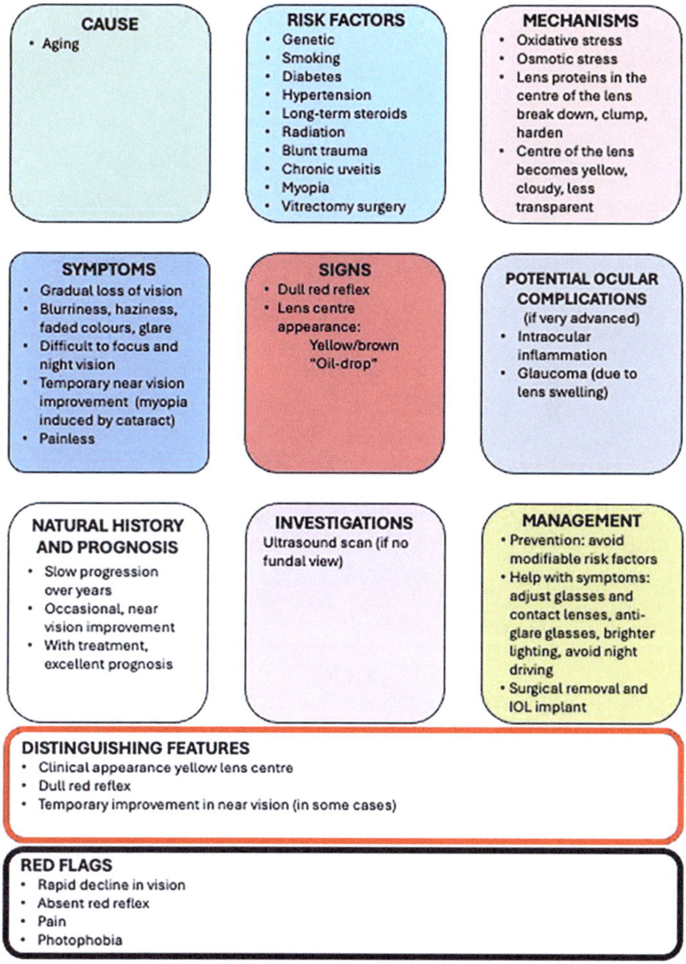

Fig. 9.2 Nucleosclerotic cataract illness script (illness script 23)

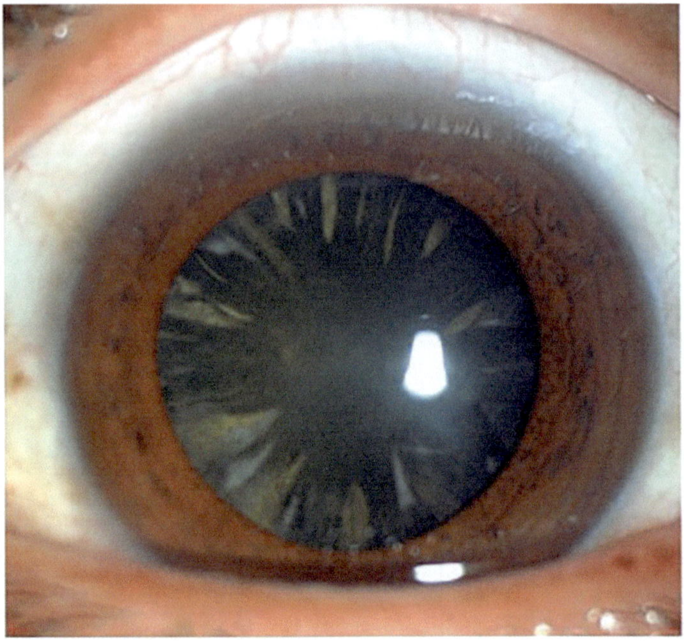

SIGNS

- "Spoke-like" pattern lens cortex opacities
- +/-retroillumination (with dilated pupil) dark shadow, opacities against retina red reflex

Fig. 9.3 Cortical cataract

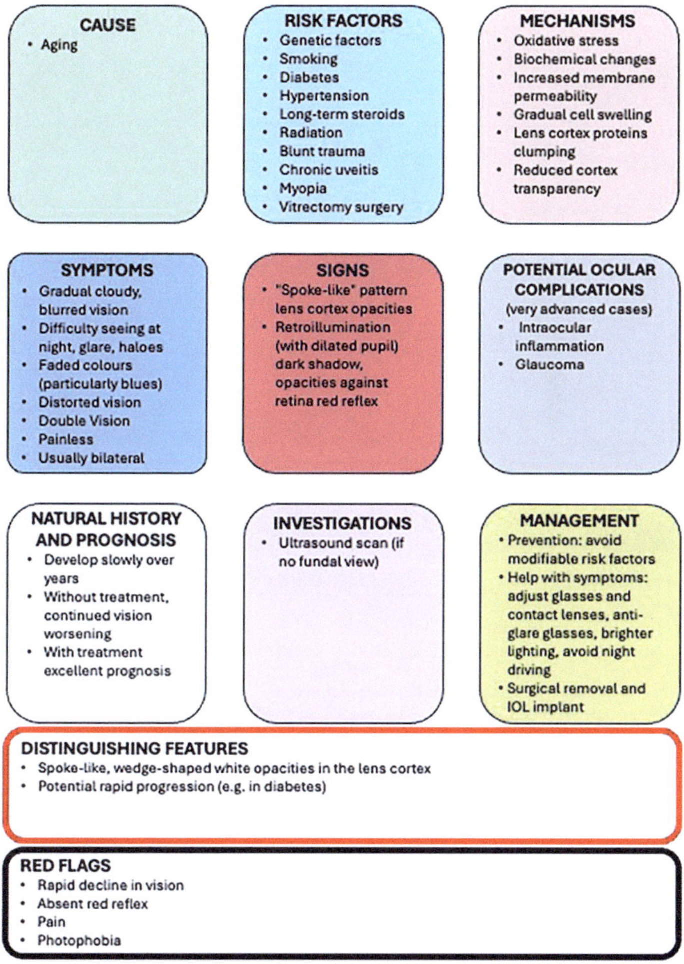

Fig. 9.4 Cortical cataract illness script (illness script 24)

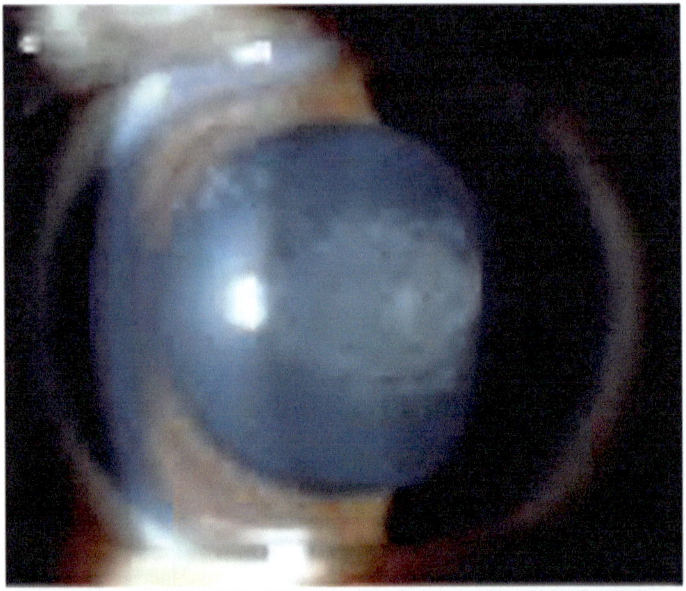

SIGNS

- "Globules", plaque in posterior part of the lens
- +/- retroillumination (with dilated pupil): dark shadow, plaque against retina red reflex

Fig. 9.5 Posterior subcapsular cataract

CAUSE
- Aging

RISK FACTORS
- Retinal dystrophies
- Glaucoma
- Genetic factors
- Smoking
- Diabetes
- Hypertension
- Long-term steroids
- Radiation
- Chronic uveitis
- Vitrectomy surgery

MECHANISMS
- Oxidative stress
- Protein clumping
- Epithelial cells dysfunction (dysplasia)
- Granular, plaque-like opacities in posterior part of the lens (block central visual axis)

SYMPTOMS
- Gradual loss of vision
- Haziness, blurriness, glare, haloes, fading colours
- Difficult near and night vision
- Painless
- Usually bilateral

SIGNS
- "Globules", plaque in posterior part of the lens
- Retroillumination (with dilated pupil): dark shadow, plaque against retina red reflex

POTENTIAL OCULAR COMPLICATIONS
(very advanced cases)
- Intraocular inflammation
- Glaucoma

NATURAL HISTORY AND PROGNOSIS
- Usually slow progression
- Occasional rapid deterioration (weeks)
- Without treatment, continue to worsen
- Prognosis excellent with cataract surgery

INVESTIGATIONS
- Ultrasound scan (if no fundal view)

MANAGEMENT
- Prevention: avoid modifiable risk factors
- Help with symptoms: adjust glasses and contact lenses, anti-glare glasses, brighter lighting, avoid night driving
- Surgical removal and IOL implant

DISTINGUISHING FEATURES
- Plaque-like or granular opacity in the posterior part of the lens
- Potential rapid progression (central location)

RED FLAGS
- Rapid decline in vision
- Absent red reflex
- Pain
- Photophobia

Fig. 9.6 Posterior subcapsular cataract illness script (illness script 25)

Table 9.1 Comparison of nucleosclerotic, cortical and posterior subcapsular cataracts illness scripts

	Nucleosclerotic cataract	Cortical cataract	Posterior subcapsular cataract
Cause	Ageing	Ageing	Ageing
Risk factors	Genetic factors Ethnicity Smoking Diabetes Hypertension Long-term use of corticosteroids Exposure to ionizing radiation (radiotherapy) Prolonged exposure to ultraviolet (UV) radiation from the sun Blunt trauma Chronic inflammation (uveitis) Myopia Eye surgery (e.g. vitrectomy) Poor diet Excessive alcohol consumption Obesity	Genetic factors Ethnicity Smoking Diabetes Hypertension Long-term use of corticosteroids Exposure to ionizing radiation (radiotherapy) Prolonged exposure to ultraviolet (UV) Blunt trauma Chronic inflammation (uveitis) Myopia Eye surgery (e.g. vitrectomy) Poor diet Excessive alcohol consumption Obesity	Retinal dystrophies Atopy Glaucoma Genetic factors Smoking Diabetes Hypertension Long-term use of corticosteroids Exposure to ionizing radiation (radiotherapy) Blunt trauma Chronic inflammation (uveitis) Myopia Eye surgery (e.g. vitrectomy) Poor diet Excessive alcohol consumption Obesity Hypoparathyroidism

Mechanisms and pathogenesis	Oxidative stress Osmotic stress Lens proteins within the central part of the lens break down, clump, harden, yellow and cloud, less transparent	Oxidative stress Biochemical changes Increased membrane permeability Gradual fibre cell damage, swelling, clumping of lens proteins in the cortex Reduced transparency	Oxidative stress Protein damage, clumping, epithelial cells dysfunction (abnormal cell migration, proliferation, dysplasia) lens posterior part granular or plaque-like opacities block the central visual axis
Symptoms	Gradual loss of vision, blurred, hazy Difficult to focus, faded colours Difficult night vision, glare, haloes Temporary improvement in near vision (myopia induced by cataract)	Gradual cloudy, blurred vision Difficulty seeing at night, glare, haloes Faded colours (particularly blues) Distorted vision Double vision	Gradual hazy, blurred vision Difficulty reading and near vision Glare, haloes Problems with night vision Yellowing, fading of colours
Signs	Yellow or brown lens Centre dull red reflex "Oil-drop" appearance	"Spoke-like" pattern lens opacities	Globules or plaque in posterior lens

(continued)

Table 9.1 (continued)

	Nucleosclerotic cataract	Cortical cataract	Posterior subcapsular cataract
Complications	Poor depth perception Monocular diplopia In very advanced cases, potentially secondary intraocular inflammation and secondary glaucoma (due to lens swelling)	Poor depth perception Monocular diplopia In very advanced cases, potentially secondary intraocular inflammation and secondary glaucoma	Poor depth perception Monocular diplopia In very advanced cases, potentially secondary intraocular inflammation and secondary glaucoma
Natural history and prognosis	Develop slowly, painlessly over many years Without treatment, progressive vision loss Occasional transient improvement in near vision (cataract-induced myopia) With treatment, excellent prognosis	Develop slowly, painlessly over many years Without treatment, continued vision worsening With treatment excellent prognosis	Develop slowly, painlessly over many years Occasionally, rapid deterioration (over weeks) Without treatment, visual function will continue to worsen Prognosis excellent with cataract surgery
Investigations	Visual acuity tests Retroillumination (with dilated pupil): dark shadow, opacity against retina red reflex Ultrasound scan (if no fundal view)	Visual acuity tests Retroillumination (with dilated pupil): dark feathered, shadow, opacity against retina red reflex Ultrasound scan (if no fundal view)	Visual acuity tests Retroillumination (with dilated pupil): dark shadow, opacity against retina red reflex Ultrasound scan (if no fundal view)

Management	Prevention, avoid modifiable risk factors Help with symptoms: adjust glasses and contact lenses, anti-glare glasses, brighter lighting, avoid night driving Surgical removal and IOL implant	Prevention, avoid modifiable risk factors Help with symptoms: adjust glasses and contact lenses, anti-glare glasses, brighter lighting, avoid night driving Surgical removal and IOL implant	Prevention, avoid modifiable risk factors Help with symptoms: adjust glasses and contact lenses, anti-glare glasses, brighter lighting, avoid night driving Surgical removal and IOL implant
Distinguishing features	Temporary improvement in near vision Clinical appearance yellow lens	Spoke-like, wedge-shaped white opacities in the cortex Potential rapid progression (e.g. in diabetes)	Feathered, plaque-like or granular opacity in the posterior lens Potential rapid progression (central location)
Red flags	Rapid decline in vision Absent red reflex Pain Photophobia	Rapid decline in vision Absent red reflex Pain Photophobia	Rapid decline in vision Absent red reflex Pain Photophobia

Glaucoma 10

Glaucoma is group of eye diseases that damage the optic nerve head, often due to increased intraocular pressure. It can lead to irreversible vision loss and blindness. Primary open angle glaucoma is a common, progressive disease where the aqueous drainage system in the anterior chamber (i.e. the trabecular meshwork) becomes clogged, leading to increased intraocular pressure that damages the optic nerve and causes peripheral irreversible vision loss (Figs. 10.1 and 10.2). It is often asymptomatic in the early stages. Acute angle closure glaucoma occurs when the iris blocks the anterior chamber angle, causing a rapid, severe rise in intraocular pressure and optic nerve head damage (Figs. 10.3 and 10.4). Congenital glaucoma is a rare but serious condition affecting infants and young children, caused by an improperly developed eye drainage system (Figs. 10.5 and 10.6).

The following illness scripts (Figs. 10.2, 10.4, and 10.6) and Table 10.1 describe and compare the elements of primary open angle glaucoma, acute angle closure glaucoma and congenital glaucoma, with emphasis on the specific distinguishing features and red flags.

M. Ugarte, *Ophthalmology Illness Scripts*,
https://doi.org/10.1007/978-3-032-31008-8_10

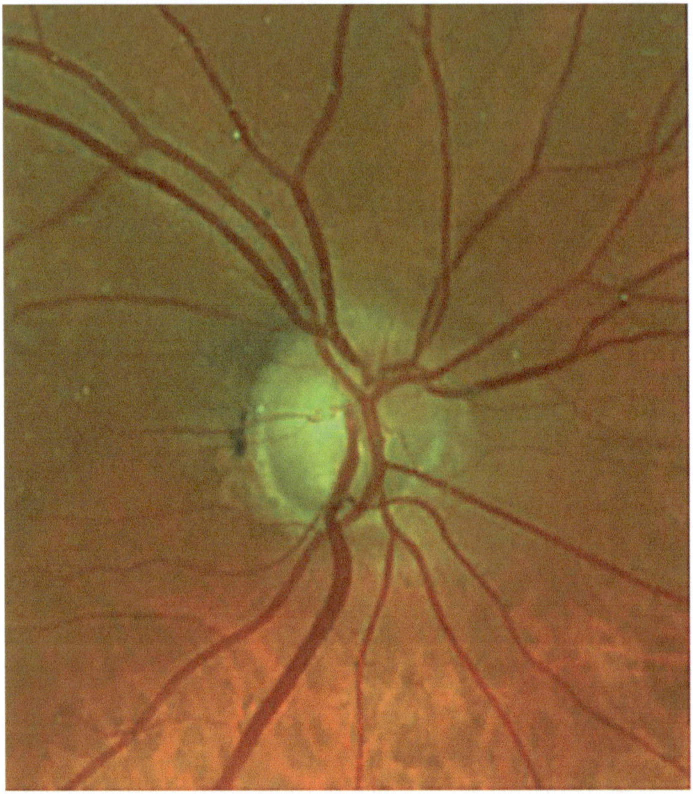

SIGNS

- High IOP (most commonly)
- Cupped optic disc
- Visual field defect

Fig. 10.1 Primary open angle glaucoma

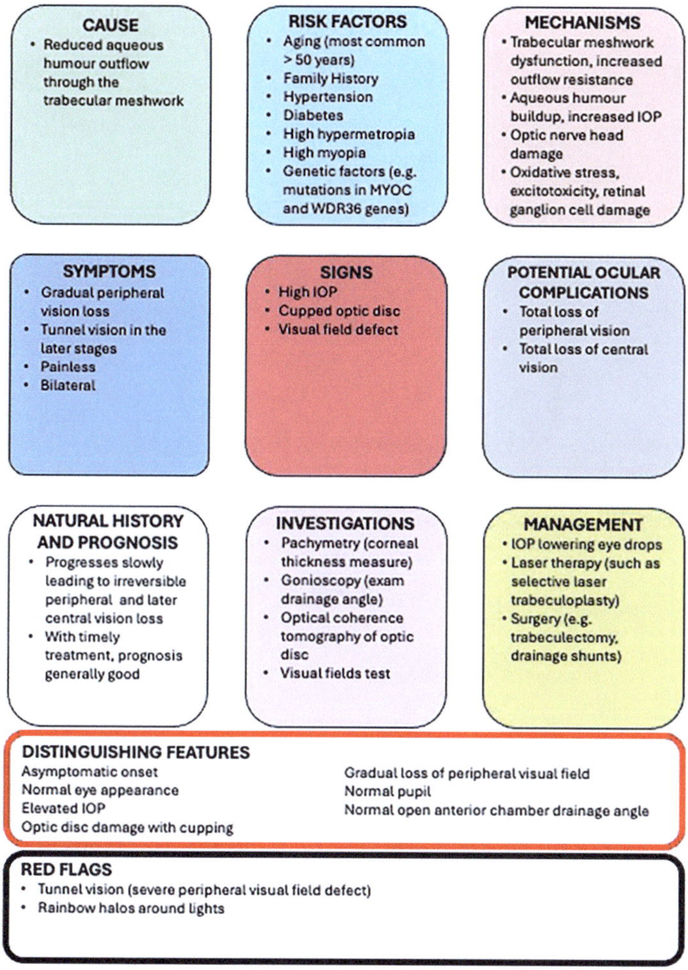

Fig. 10.2 Primary open angle glaucoma illness script (illness script 26)

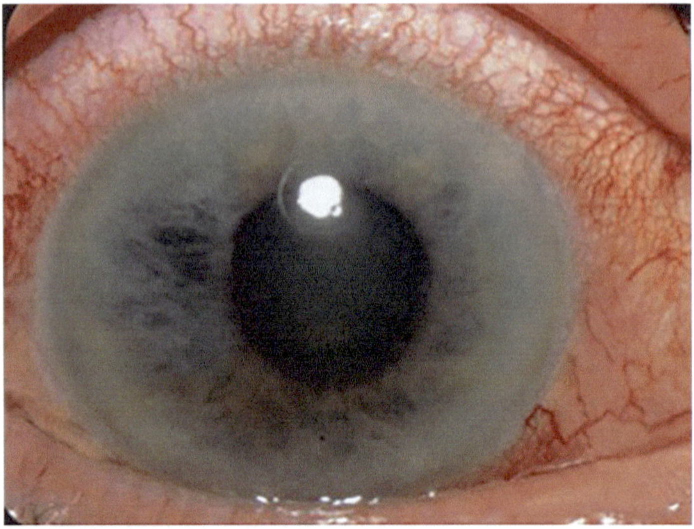

SIGNS

- Red eye
- Corneal haze
- Fixed, mid-dilated pupil
- Very raised IOP (eyeball feels hard)

Fig. 10.3 Acute angle closure glaucoma

CAUSE
- Blockage of the anterior chamber drainage angle by the iris

RISK FACTORS
- Aging
- Female
- Asian
- Narrow angles
- Thickened lens
- Family history
- Hypermetropia
- Pupil-dilating agents
- Intraocular tumours
- Trauma

MECHANISMS
- Pupil block after pupil dilatation
- Iris bulge forwards
- Trabecular meshwork block
- Aqueous humour drainage interruption
- Severe rise of IOP

SYMPTOMS
- Sudden onset
- Usually one eye
- Intense eye pain
- Blurred vision
- Rainbow-coloured circles around lights
- Headache
- Nausea, vomiting
- Generally unwell

SIGNS
- Red eye
- Corneal haze
- Fixed, mid-dilated pupil
- Very raised IOP (eyeball feels hard)

POTENTIAL OCULAR COMPLICATIONS
- Corneal decompensation
- Chronic angle closure glaucoma
- Cataract
- Central or branch retinal vein occlusion

NATURAL HISTORY AND PROGNOSIS
- Acute onset
- Possible recurrences
- Delayed treatment can lead to blindness
- With immediate, timely treatment, prognosis good

INVESTIGATIONS
- Gonioscopy (exam drainage angle)
- Ultrasound scan to assess posterior segment

MANAGEMENT
(medical emergency)
- Acetazolamide IV
- Pilocarpine eye drops
- Steroid eye drops
- IOP lowering eye drops
- Analgesia
- Anti-emetic
- Laser peripheral iridotomy (both eyes, prophylaxis fellow eye)

DISTINGUISHING FEATURES
- Severe eye pain/headache
- Haloes around lights
- Very high IOP
- Shallow anterior chamber

Usually one eye
Conjunctival injection
Hazy oedematous cornea
Closed anterior chamber angle

Sudden blurred vision
Nausea and vomiting
Fixed, mid-dilated pupil

RED FLAGS
- Sudden, severe eye pain
- Seeing haloes around lights
- Headache, nausea, vomiting
- Fixed, mid-dilated pupil

Fig. 10.4 Acute angle closure glaucoma illness script (illness script 27)

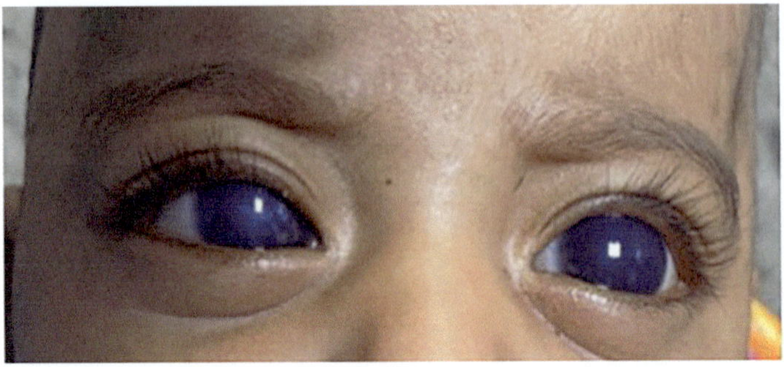

SIGNS

- Eye size enlarged (buphthalmos)
- Squint
- Cornea cloudy or opacfied
- Cornea Descemet's membrane breaks (Haab´s striae)
- Nystagmus

Fig. 10.5 Congenital glaucoma

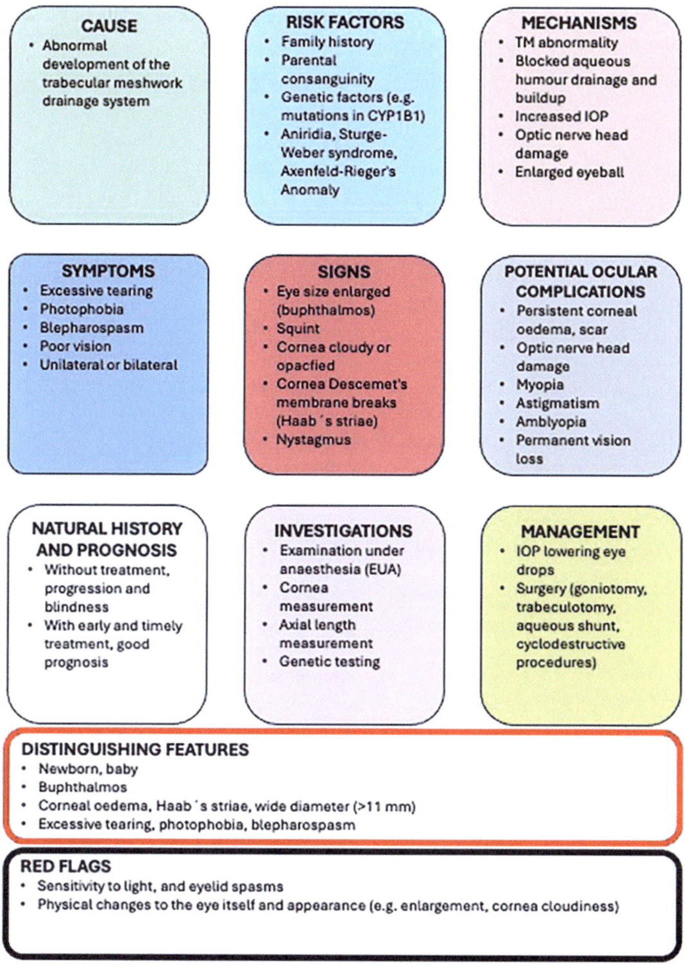

Fig. 10.6 Congenital glaucoma illness script (illness script 28)

Table 10.1 Comparison of primary open angle glaucoma, acute angle closure glaucoma and congenital glaucoma illness scripts

	Primary open angle glaucoma	Acute angle closure glaucoma	Congenital glaucoma
Cause	Reduced aqueous humour outflow through the trabecular meshwork	Blockage of the anterior chamber drainage angle by the iris	Abnormal development of the trabecular meshwork drainage system before birth
Risk factors	Ageing (most common >50 years) Ethnicity: African, Asian, Hispanic descent Family history Medical conditions; high blood pressure, diabetes High hypermetropia High myopia Elevated intraocular pressure Genetic factors (e.g. mutations in MYOC and WDR36 genes)	Ageing Female Asian Shallow anterior chambers Narrower drainage angles Plateau iris Thickened crystalline lens Stress Family history of glaucoma Hypermetropia Anticholinergic, sympathomimetic, serotonergic Pupil-dilating agents Intraocular tumours History of trauma	Family history of congenital glaucoma Genetic factors (e.g. mutations in CYP1B1) Parental consanguinity Syndromes: aniridia, Sturge-Weber syndrome, Axenfeld-Rieger's Anomaly

(continued)

Table 10.1 (continued)

	Primary open angle glaucoma	Acute angle closure glaucoma	Congenital glaucoma
Mechanisms and pathogenesis	Trabecular meshwork dysfunction with increased resistance Build-up of aqueous humour Increased intraocular pressure Optic nerve damage	Pupil block after pupil dilatation Posterior segment pathology (e.g. choroidal effusion or posterior segment tumours) Forward shift of the lens-iris diaphragm	TM doesn't form correctly Blocks drainage Fluid build-up and increased IOP Amage to the optic nerve head
	Inadequate blood supply to the optic nerve Oxidative stress Cytokine dysregulation Excitotoxicity, damage to RGCs	The iris bulges forward and blocks the trabecular meshwork Aqueous drainage blockage Raised intraocular pressure Cornea, retina, optic nerve head damage	
Symptoms	Painless Gradual peripheral vision loss Tunnel vision in the later stages	Sudden onset Usually one eye Intense eye pain Red eye Blurred vision Rainbow-colored circles around lights Headache Nausea and vomiting Generally unwell	Excessive tearing Photophobia Blepharospasm Poor vision Unilateral or bilateral

(continued)

Table 10.1 (continued)

	Primary open angle glaucoma	Acute angle closure glaucoma	Congenital glaucoma
Signs	High IOP Cupped optic disc Visual field defect	Fixed, mid-dilated pupil Corneal haze	Cloudy or opacified cornea Enlargement of eye size (buphthalmos) Breaks in cornea Descemet's membrane (Haab's striae) Squint
Complications	Loss of peripheral vision Loss of central vision Complete blindness	Corneal decompensation Cataract formation Fixed dilated pupil Chronic angle closure glaucoma Recurrent episodes Central or branch retinal vein occlusion	Corneal scarring Persistent corneal oedema Optic nerve head damage Myopia Astigmatism Amblyopia Permanent vision loss
		Peripheral anterior synechiae Damage to the anterior chamber angle	
		Aqueous misdirection syndrome	

(continued)

Table 10.1 (continued)

	Primary open angle glaucoma	Acute angle closure glaucoma	Congenital glaucoma
Natural history and prognosis	Untreated, progresses slowly over many years, leading to irreversible peripheral vision loss and potentially central vision loss and blindness With treatment, prognosis generally good, delay or stop disease progression The speed progresses is variable African descendants may experience faster progression and more refractory case	Acute onset With immediate, timely treatment, prognosis is generally good Delayed treatment can lead to permanent vision loss or blindness	Without treatment, progression and blindness Early and timely treatment is essential to preserve a child's vision and prevent blindness

(continued)

Table 10.1 (continued)

	Primary open angle glaucoma	Acute angle closure glaucoma	Congenital glaucoma
Investisgations	Slit-lamp biomicroscopy Measuring intraocular pressure Pachymetry (measure corneal thickness) Gonioscopy (examine drainage angle) Funduscopy (examine optic disc) OCT (optic disc assessment) Visual fields test using perimetry	Slit-lamp examination (assess anterior chamber) Tonometry (measure intraocular pressure) Gonioscopy (assess anterior chamber angle) Visual fields (perimetry) Optic nerve head assessment	Examination under anaesthesia Corneal measurements Anterior segment exam Tonometry Fundus and optic disc imaging Axial length measurement Genetic testing Cycloplegic refraction
Management	IOP lowering eye drops Laser therapy (such as selective laser Trabeculoplasty Surgery (drainage shunts or trabeculoplasty)	Laser peripheral iridotomy Cataract surgery Emergency medical therapy: Acetazolamide IV Pilocarpine eye drops Analgesia Anti-emetic	Eye drops to lower IOP often the first line of treatment used as a temporary measure Surgery: Goniotomy Trabeculotomy Aqueous shunt devices Cyclodestructive procedures

(continued)

Table 10.1 (continued)

	Primary open angle glaucoma	Acute angle closure glaucoma	Congenital glaucoma
Distinguishing features	Asymptomatic onset Gradual loss of vision (peripheral visual field) Normal eye appearance Normal pupil Elevated IOP Optic disc damage Visual field defect Open anterior chamber angle	Severe eye pain or headache Usually one eye Sudden blurred vision Haloes around lights Red eye: conjunctival injection, ciliary flush Nausea and vomiting Very high intraocular pressure Hazy oedematous cornea Fixed, mid-dilated pupil Shallow anterior chamber Closed anterior chamber angle	Buphthalmos Corneal oedema and opacity Corneal Haab's striae Abnormally wide corneal diameter (>11 mm) Excessive tearing Photophobia Blepharospasm Optic disc damage Progressive myopia Nystagmus in some cases
Red flags	Subtle at first Tunnel vision Rainbow halos around lights	Sudden, severe eye pain Redness Blurred/cloudy vision Seeing halos around lights Headache, nausea, vomiting Fixed, mid-dilated pupil	Excessive tearing, sensitivity to light, and eyelid spasms. Other key signs involve physical changes to the eye itself, such as enlargement and cloudiness

11 Retinal Vascular Occlusions (Branch and Central, Vein and Artery Occlusions)

A retinal vascular (artery or vein) occlusion usually presents by a sudden, painless loss or vision in one eye. Key features identified during fundal examination include signs depending on whether a central or branch retinal vessel has been affected. In a retinal vein occlusion, blood and fluid leaks into the retinal tissue causing haemorrhages and macular oedema (Figs. 11.1, 11.2, 11.3, and 11.4). In a retinal artery occlusion, oxygen-rich blood supply is cut off and the retina appears white (Figs. 11.5, 11.6, 11.7, and 11.8).

The following illness scripts (Figs. 11.2, 11.4, and 11.6) and Table 11.1 describe and compare the elements of branch and central retinal vein and artery occlusions, highlighting the specific distinguishing features and red flags.

M. Ugarte, *Ophthalmology Illness Scripts*,
https://doi.org/10.1007/978-3-032-31008-8_11

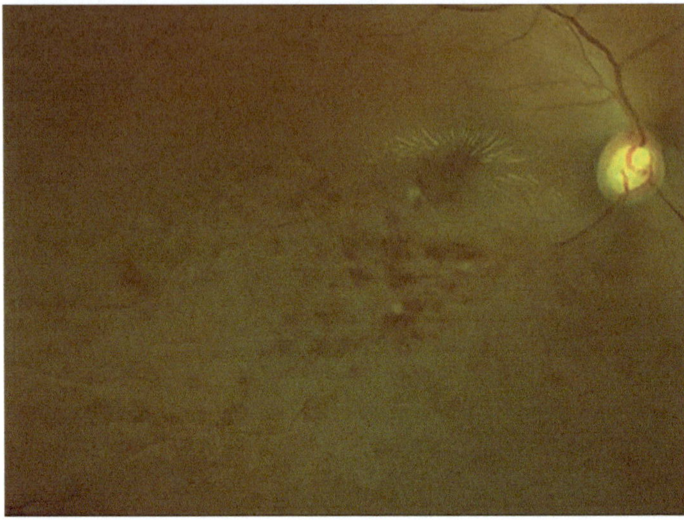

SIGNS

(funduscopy)

- Retinal haemorrhages (dot, blot, flame-shaped) in segmental distribution
- Venous congestion
- Retinal oedema
- Retina exudates
- +/- cotton-wool spots
- Attenuated arteries

Fig. 11.1 Branch retinal vein occlusion

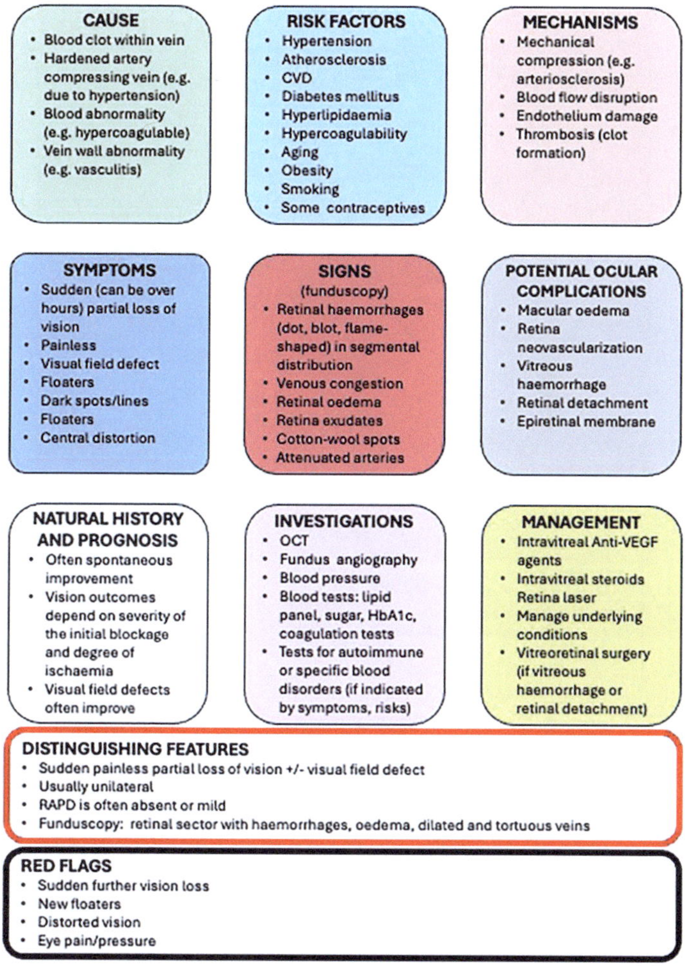

Fig. 11.2 Branch retinal vein occlusion illness script (illness script 29)

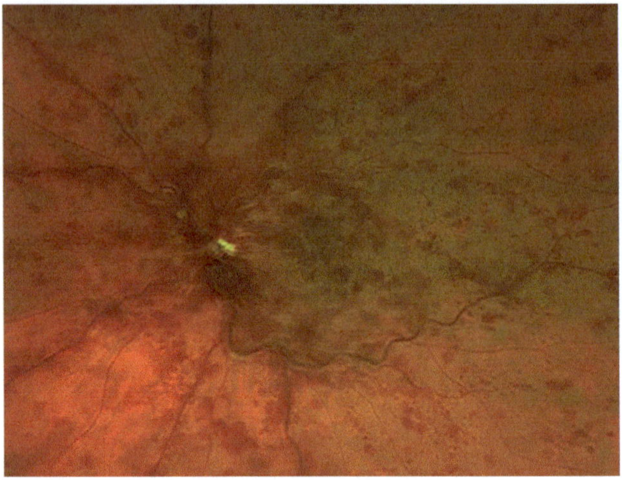

SIGNS

- Retina haemorrhages in 4 quadrants
- Dilated, tortuous veins
- +/- macular oedema
- +/- cotton-wool spots
- +/- swollen optic disc)black arrow)
- +/- RAPD

Fig. 11.3 Central retinal vein occlusion

CAUSE
- Blood clot
- Hardened artery compress central retinal vein
- Abnormality of blood (hypercoagulability)
- Abnormality of vein wall (vasculitis)
- Vein compression from high IOP

RISK FACTORS
- Hypertension
- Hyperlipidaemia
- Diabetes
- Aging
- CVD, heart disease
- Coagulopathies
- Glaucoma
- Smoking
- Systemic vasculitis
- Some contraceptives

MECHANISMS
- Anatomical compression
- Thrombosis
- Increased capillary pressure and vascular permeability
- Fluid leakage
- Ischemia
- Cytokines release
- Neovascularisation

SYMPTOMS
- Sudden loss of vision, blurriness affecting the whole visual field
- Painless
- Floaters
- Distorted vision
- Unilateral

SIGNS
- Retina haemorrhages in 4 quadrants
- Dilated, tortuous veins
- +/- macular oedema
- +/- cotton-wool spots
- +/- swollen optic disc
- +/- RAPD

POTENTIAL OCULAR COMPLICATIONS
- Macular oedema
- Retina +/- optic disc neovascularisation
- Neovascular glaucoma
- Vitreous haemorrhage
- Retinal detachment
- Optic disc collaterals

NATURAL HISTORY AND PROGNOSIS
(depends on degree of ischaemia, initial vision)
- Non-ischemic CRVO, 50% improvement

INVESTIGATIONS
- OCT
- Fundus angiography
- Blood pressure
- Blood test: FBC, ESR, CRP, lipids, HbA1c, thyroid function
- Tests for vasculitis, kidney disease, ECG (based on signs and risk factors)

MANAGEMENT
- Underlying conditions
- Intravitreal anti-VEGF agents
- Intravitreal steroids
- Retina laser
- Vitreoretinal surgery (if vitreous haemorrhage, retinal detachment)

DISTINGUISHING FEATURES
- Sudden vision loss, entire visual field defect
- Affects all four quadrants on funduscopy
- Painless
- RAPD present in severe, ischemic CRVO

RED FLAGS
- Sudden severe further vision loss
- New floaters
- Distorted vision
- Eye pain

Fig. 11.4 Central retinal vein occlusion illness script (illness script 30)

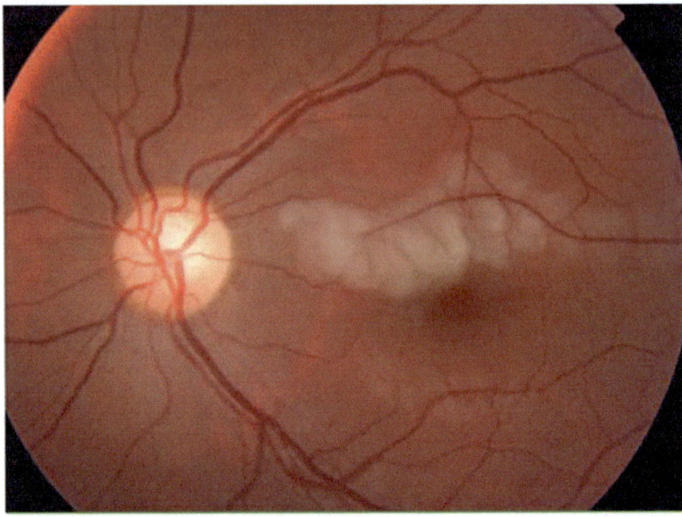

SIGNS

- Pale retina in a sector
- +/- arteriole embolus
- +/- arterial wall inflammation

Fig. 11.5 Branch retinal artery occlusion

CAUSE
- Blood clot (embolus)
- Vasculitis
- Clotting disorders
- Vasospasm
- Atherosclerosis
- Infections

RISK FACTORS
- Hypertension
- Hyperlipidaemia
- Diabetes
- Aging
- CVD, heart disease
- Coagulopathies
- Glaucoma
- Smoking
- Systemic vasculitis

MECHANISMS
- Embolism (e.g. cholesterol plaques, fibrin/platelets, calcific)
- Vasospasm
- Artery wall inflammation
- Ischaemia

SYMPTOMS
- Sudden partial loss of vision
- Painless
- Unilateral
- Fluctuating vision loss (amaurosis fugax)
- Asymptomatic (depending on location of blocked arteriole)

SIGNS
(funduscopy)
- Pale retina
- +/- Arteriole embolus
- +/- Arterial wall inflammation

POTENTIAL OCULAR COMPLICATIONS
- Retinal atrophy
- Retina neovascularisation (rare)
- Increased risk systemic vascular events (e.g. stroke, heart attack)

NATURAL HISTORY AND PROGNOSIS
- Temporary occlusions excellent prognosis
- Permanent occlusions, visual field defects permanent

INVESTIGATIONS
- OCT
- Fundus angiography
- Blood pressure
- Blood test: FBC, ESR, CRP, HbA1c, lipids,
- Test for vasculitis, clotting disorders (based on signs and risk factors)

MANAGEMENT
- Referral to stroke unit
- Underlying systemic condition
- Thrombolysis (not proven effect)
- Retina laser +/- intravitreal anti-VEGF agents (if retina neovascularisation)

DISTINGUISHING FEATURES
- Sudden visual loss in a sector
- Unilateral
- Painless
- On funduscopy, retina sector whitening, +/- arteriole embolus, +/- arterial wall inflammation

RED FLAGS
- Associated systemic symptoms
- Further reduction in vision
- Floates

Fig. 11.6 Branch retinal artery occlusion illness script (illness script 31)

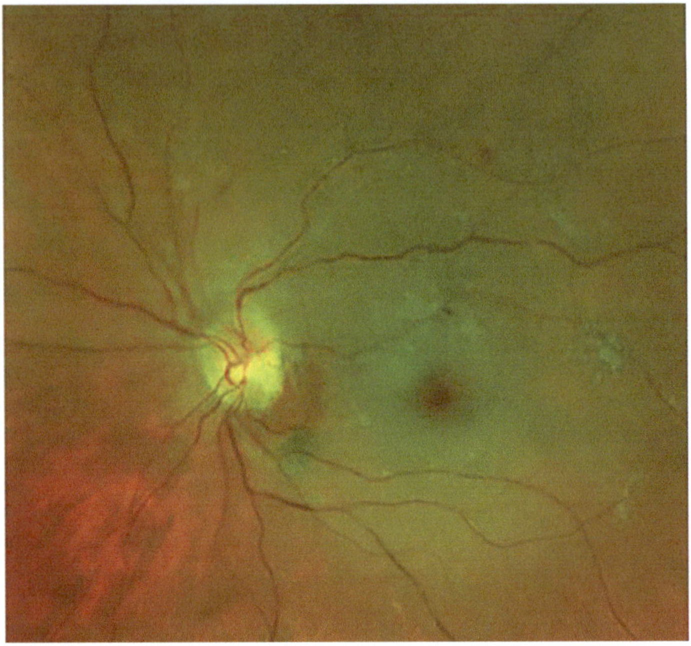

SIGNS:

- Retina whitening
- Cherry-red spot
- Arterioles attenuation
- +/- nasal macula perfused if clilioretinal artery present and patent
- +/-embolus
- +/-arterial segmented blood flow ("boxcarring)
- Relative afferent pupillary defect

Fig. 11.7 Central retinal artery occlusion

CAUSE
- Embolus (e.g. fibrin, cholesterol, calcium)
- Atherosclerosis
- Inflammation of artery wall (e.g. giant cell arteritis)
- Compression

RISK FACTORS
- Aging
- Male
- Smoking
- Hypertension
- Hyperlipidaemia
- Diabetes
- CVD, heart disease
- Coagulopathies
- Vasculitis (e.g. GCA)
- Glaucoma

MECHANISMS
- Embolism
- Vasospasm
- Artery compression
- Ischaemia

SYMPTOMS
- Sudden complete loss of vision
- Painless
- Unilateral
- Fluctuating vision loss (amaurosis fugax)

SIGNS:
- Relative afferent pupillary defect
- Retina whitening
- Cherry-red spot
- Arterioles attenuation
- +/-embolus
- +/-arterial segmented blood flow ("boxcarring)

POTENTIAL OCULAR COMPLICATIONS
- Retinal atrophy
- Optic disc atrophy
- Retina +/- optic disc neovascularisation
- Vitreous haemorrhage
- Neovascular glaucoma

NATURAL HISTORY AND PROGNOSIS
- Approximately, 90% poor vision
- Factors Influencing: aetiology, cilioretinal artery involvement
- Increased risk of systemic cardiovascular events

INVESTIGATIONS
- OCT
- Fundus angiography
- Blood pressure
- Blood tests: FBC, lipids, HbA1c, ESR, CRP
- Tests for vasculitis, clotting disorders (based on signs and risk factors)

MANAGEMENT
- Eye massage
- IOP lowering
- Acetazolamide iv
- Thrombolysis (limited effect)
- Referral to stroke unit
- Intravitreal anti-VEGF and/or retina laser if new vessels

DISTINGUISHING FEATURES
- Sudden complete loss of vision
- Unilateral
- Fundal examination: "cherry-red spot"
- Arterial attenuation, +/- embolus, "box carring"

Painless
RAPD typically present
Retinal whitening
History of amaurosis fugax

RED FLAGS
- Associated systemic symptoms (e.g. TIA, GCA)
- Eye pain

Fig. 11.8 Central retinal artery occlusion illness script (illness script 32)

Table 11.1 Comparison of branch, central vein and artery occlusions illness scripts

	Branch retinal vein occlusion	Central retinal vein occlusion	Branch retinal artery occlusion	Central retinal artery occlusion
Cause	Blood clot Hardened artery compressing a vein (hypertension) Abnormality of blood (hypercoagulability) Abnormality of vein wall (vasculitis)	Blood clot Hardened artery compress vein Abnormality of blood (hypercoagulability) Abnormality of vein wall (vasculitis) Compression from high IOP	Blood clot (embolus) Inflammation of vessel wall (vasculitis) Blood clotting disorders Vasospasm Infections Atherosclerosis Autoimmune Trauma, surgery	Clot embolus (fibrin, cholesterol, calcium) Atherosclerosis Inflammation of artery wall (e.g. giant cell arteritis) Clotting disorders Trauma Compression from masses

Risk factors	Hypertension Atherosclerosis Carotid artery disease Diabetes Mellitus Hyperlipidaemia Cardiovascular disease Heart disease (e.g. AF) Stroke history Obesity & high BMI Hypercoagulability (e.g. antiphospholipid syndrome) Ageing Oral contraceptives & IV drug Smoking	Hypertension Atherosclerosis Hyperlipidaemia Diabetes Hyperviscosity Ageing Oral contraceptives Cardiovascular disease Heart disease (e.g. AF) Coagulation abnormalities Glaucoma Smoking Systemic vasculitis	Carotid artery disease Ischaemic heart disease Hypertension Hyperlipidaemia Cardiovascular disease Heart disease Diabetes Smoking Ageing Atherosclerosis Obesity Oral contraceptives & IV drug Hypercoagulable state	Hypertension Atherosclerosis Hyperlipidaemia Diabetes Hyperviscosity Cardiovascular disease Carotid artery disease Heart disease (e.g. AF) Coagulation abnormalities Raised intraocular ocular pressure (e.g. glaucoma) Smoking Systemic vasculitis (e.g. GCA) Ageing Male

(continued)

Table 11.1 (continued)

	Branch retinal vein occlusion	Central retinal vein occlusion	Branch retinal artery occlusion	Central retinal artery occlusion
Mechanisms and pathogenesis	Mechanical compression Arteriosclerosis Shared sheath Compression Blood flow disruption Turbulence Endothelial damage Thrombosis (clot formation)	Anatomical compression Thrombosis (clot) Increase pressure in capillaries Fluid leakage (e.g. macular oedema) Ischemia Release inflammatory cytokines (e.g. VEGF, IL-6, IL-8) Damage vessels, increase permeability Neovascularization	Embolism Cholesterol plaques Fibrin/platelet clots Calcific emboli Other emboli Vasospasm Artery compression Ischaemia	Embolism Thrombosis Vasospasm Vascular compression Vasculitis Narrow or block central retinal artery entering the optic nerve Stop blood flow Sudden ischaemia
Symptoms	Sudden (can be over hours) painless partial loss of vision in one eye Dark spots/lines Floaters Visual field defect	Sudden, painless vision loss/blurriness Floaters Distorted vision	Sudden, painless partial loss of vision in one eye Fluctuating vision loss (amaurosis fugax) as embolus (e.g. fibrin-platelet) passes through circulation Can be asymptomatic (depending on location of blocked arteriole)	Sudden, painless permanent total loss of vision in one eye (seconds to minutes) Fluctuating loss of vision (amaurosis fugax) as embolus (e.g. fibrin-platelet) passes through the retinal circulation

Signs	Retinal haemorrhages (dot, blot, and flame-shaped) in segmental distribution Retinal oedema Venous congestion (stasis) Retina exudates Retina ischaemia Cotton-wool spots Attenuated arterial vessel calibre	Retina haemorrhages widespread (four quadrants) Macular oedema Cotton-wool spots Dilated veins	Pale retina	Relative afferent pupillary defect Pale retina Cherry-red spot Arterioles attenuation Emboli Arteries segmented blood flow, "box carring"
Complications	Macular oedema Neovascularization Retinal detachment Vitreous haemorrhage Epiretinal membrane	Macular oedema Retina, optic disc new vessels Neovascular glaucoma: new vessels block drainage angle, cause very high IOP Vitreous haemorrhage Retinal detachment	Permanent vision loss (either partial or complete) Retinal neovascularization (rare) Retinal atrophy Increased risk systemic vascular events (e.g. stroke, heart attack)	Permanent blindness New blood vessels on the iris (neovascular glaucoma) or retina (proliferative retinopathy) Optic atrophy Vitreous haemorrhage Stroke/heart attack increased risk

(continued)

Table 11.1 (continued)

	Branch retinal vein occlusion	Central retinal vein occlusion	Branch retinal artery occlusion	Central retinal artery occlusion
Natural history and prognosis	Spontaneous improvement is common Vision outcomes depend on the severity of the initial blockage Vision loss mainly due to macular oedema Bleeding into the eye Visual field defects often improve or stabilize	Spontaneous improvement: 50% non-ischaemic CRVO Prognosis based on initial vision Vision 6/6 or better: vision likely to stay the same or improve Vision 6/24–6/60: can improve, stay same, or worsen Vision <6/60: usually no improvement	Temporary occlusions excellent prognosis (100%, 6/12 or better) Permanent occlusions less certain Spontaneous improvement: up to 80% good vision (6/12 or better) over time if fovea not involved Visual field defects typically permanent	Limited spontaneous recovery Around 90% of patients end up with poor vision (6/120 or worse) Factors influencing outcome Time to treatment Aetiology Cilioretinal artery involvement Systemic risk of stroke and ischemic heart disease

Investigations	Optical coherence tomography Fluorescein angiography Optical coherence tomography angiography Blood pressure Blood tests: lipid panel, blood sugar, coagulation tests Tests for autoimmune conditions or specific blood disorders (if indicated by symptoms)	Optical coherence tomography Fluorescein angiography Optical coherence tomography angiography Blood pressure Blood sugar, HbA1c, lipids, FBC, ESR, CRP Thyroid function tests Screens for inflammation (vasculitis), kidney disease and ECG (if indicated by symptoms)	Optical coherence tomography Fluorescein angiography Visual field test Blood tests: FBC, lipid profile, fasting glucose/HbA1c, ESR/CRP, clotting studies Carotid ultrasound ECG Brain MRI/MRA Referral to stroke unit	Optical coherence tomography Fluorescein angiography Visual field test Blood tests: FBC, lipid profile, fasting glucose/HbA1c, ESR/CRP, clotting studies Carotid ultrasound ECG Brain MRI/MRA Referral to stroke unit

(continued)

Table 11.1 (continued)

	Branch retinal vein occlusion	Central retinal vein occlusion	Branch retinal artery occlusion	Central retinal artery occlusion
Management	Intravitreal injections Anti-VEGF agents Corticosteroid (e.g. Dexamethasone implant, Ozurdex) Laser treatment Focal/grid laser Pan retinal photocoagulation (PRP) Management of underlying conditions	Intravitreal injections Anti-VEGF agents Corticosteroid (e.g. Dexamethasone implant, Ozurdex) Laser treatment Focal/grid laser Pan retinal photocoagulation Management of underlying conditions	Eye massage Intraocular pressure lowering Acetazolamide Thrombolysis (clot-busting drugs, laser therapy) (limited effectiveness) Intravitreal anti-VEGF and/or retina laser if neovascularization	Acute treatment Dilate arteriole to permit embolus pass more distally (worth try in 24 h) (limited benefit) Lower IOP Intravenous acetazolamide Ocular massage Paracentesis Rebreathe into a paper bag May benefit from immediate anticoagulant or antiplatelet (e.g. aspirin) if not contraindicated Management of underlying condition and complications Intravitreal anti-VEGF and/or retina laser if neovascularization

Distinguishing features	Sudden painless partial loss of vision or visual field defect, often in 1 eye Affects a sector (wedge) of the retina on fundus examination: haemorrhages, retina oedema, dilated, tortuous veins RAPD is often absent or mild	Sudden painless vision loss or entire visual field defect Affects all four quadrants on fundus exam Optic disc oedema RAPD present in severe, ischemic CRVO	Sudden painless unilateral partial visual loss in a sector. On funduscopic examination, retina whitening, embolus can be seen	Sudden, painless, unilateral loss of vision, often complete RAPD typically present Fundal examination: "cherry-red spot" at the macula Retinal whitening Arterial attenuation Box carring Emboli may be seen History of amaurosis fugax
Red flags	Sudden severe vision loss New floaters Distorted vision Eye pain/pressure	Sudden severe vision loss New floaters Distorted vision Eye pain/pressure	Associated symptoms (>55) New headaches, jaw pain (claudication), scalp tenderness, fatigue	Associated symptoms (>55) Stroke TIA GCA

Diabetic Retinopathy 12

Diabetic retinopathy is a progressive microvascular disease resulting from chronic high blood sugar. It results in damaged capillary walls, leakage, and gradual closure of retinal blood vessels. It is classified by the stage of the disease, non-proliferative to proliferative forms. The latter is the advanced sight-threatening stage with the presence of new abnormal blood vessels (neovascularization). Retinal microaneurysms are one of the hallmarks of diabetic retinopathy, which can help distinguish it from other retinopathies (e.g. hypertensive retinopathy). Typically, bilateral, affecting both eyes over time (Figs. 12.1, 12.2, 12.3, 12.4, 12.5, and 12.6).

The following illness scripts (Figs. 12.2, 12.4, and 12.6) and Table 12.1 describe and compare the elements of diabetic maculopathy, non-proliferative and proliferative diabetic retinopathy, highlighting their distinguishing features and red flags.

M. Ugarte, *Ophthalmology Illness Scripts*,
https://doi.org/10.1007/978-3-032-31008-8_12

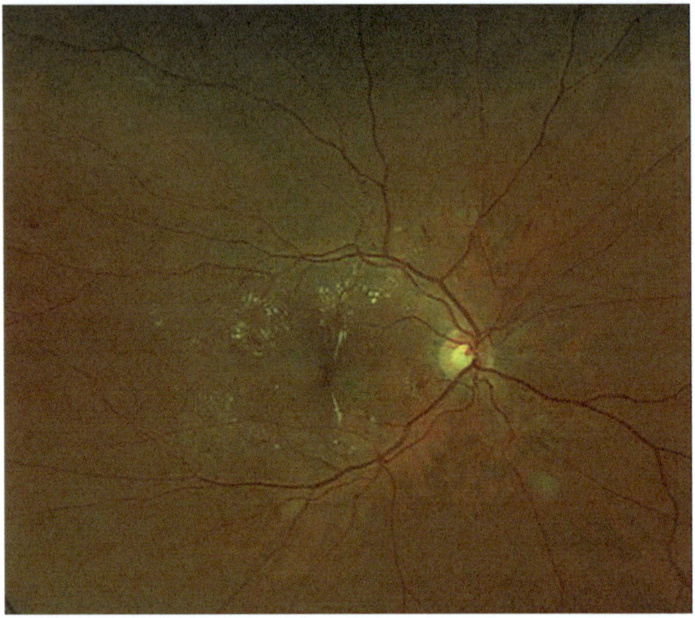

SIGNS

- Retinal microaneurysms
- Haemorrhages
- Exudates
- Retinal oedema
- Microvascular abnormalities

Fig. 12.1 Diabetic maculopathy

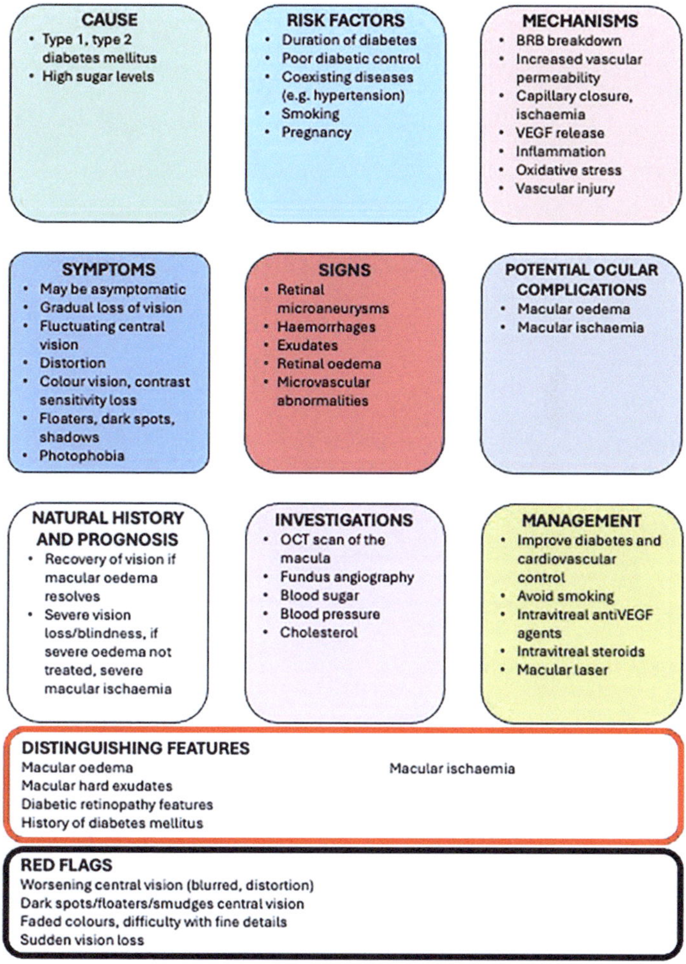

Fig. 12.2 Diabetic maculopathy illness script (illness script 33)

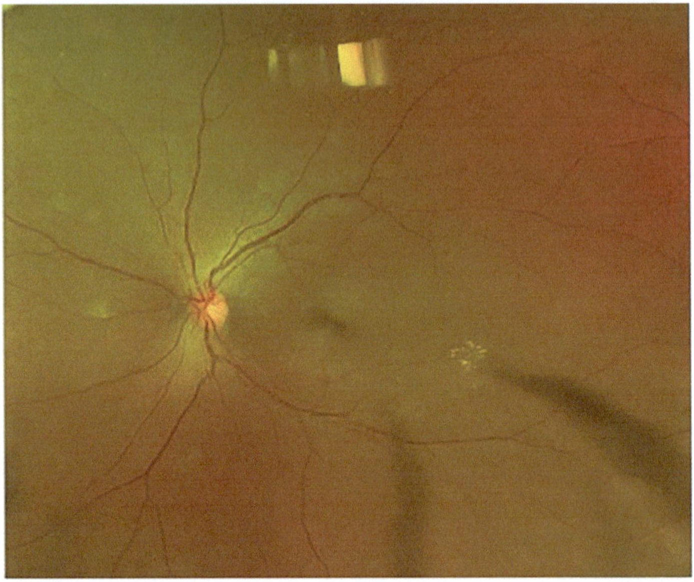

SIGNS

- Retinal microaneurysms
- Haemorrhages
- Exudates
- Retinal oedema
- Microvascular abnormalities

Fig. 12.3 Non-proliferative diabetic retinopathy

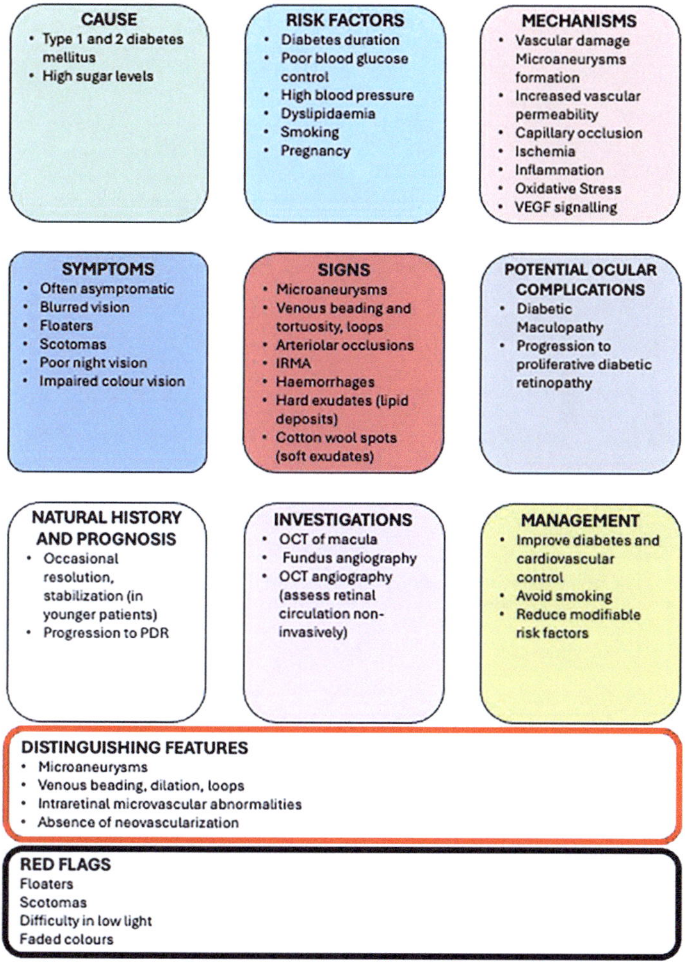

Fig. 12.4 Non-proliferative diabetic retinopathy illness script (illness script 34)

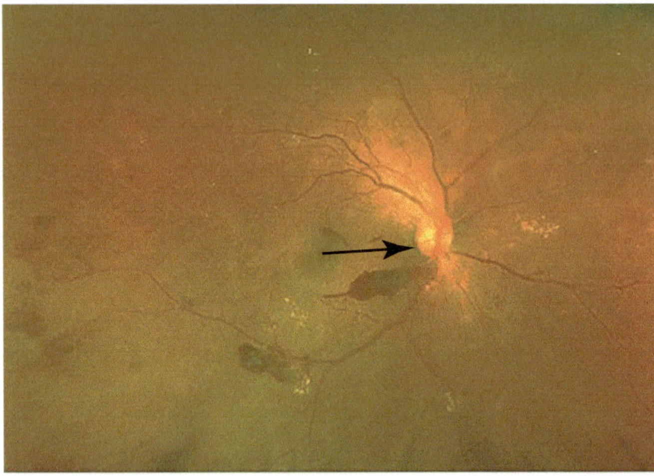

SIGNS

- In addition to signs of NPDR
- New vessels on the optic disc (NVD) (black arrow) or retina elsewhere (NVE)
- +/- neuroretina traction

Fig. 12.5 Proliferative diabetic retinopathy

CAUSE
- Type 1 and 2 diabetes mellitus
- High sugar levels
- Hypoxia

RISK FACTORS
- Duration of diabetes
- Young age at diagnosis
- Poor diabetic control
- Cardiovascular comorbidities
- Smoking
- Pregnancy
- Genetics and ethnicity

MECHANISMS
- Vascular damage
- Vascular closure Ischemia
- Hypoxia
- Inflammation
- Oxidative stress
- Neovascularization
- Excitotoxicity
- MicroRNAs changes

SYMPTOMS
- Sometimes asymptomatic
- Floaters
- Flashing lights
- Sudden loss of vision

SIGNS
- In addition to signs of NPDR
- New vessels on the optic disc (NVD) or retina elsewhere (NVE)
- Neuroretina traction

POTENTIAL OCULAR COMPLICATIONS
- Preretinal haemorrhage
- Vitreous haemorrhage
- Tractional retinal detachment
- Neovascular glaucoma

NATURAL HISTORY AND PROGNOSIS
- Treatment (retina laser +/- intravitreal anti-VEGF agents) may maintain good vision
- Poor prognosis in cases with NVD, NVE with haemorrhage
- Potentially blinding

INVESTIGATIONS
- OCT scan of the macula
- Fundus angiography
- Blood sugar
- Blood pressure control
- Ultrasound B scan (if no fundal view)

MANAGEMENT
- Retina laser (i.e. PRP)
- Intravitreal anti-VEGF agents
- Improve diabetes, cardiovascular risk factors
- Vitreoretinal surgery (if vitreous haemorrhage, retinal detachment)

DISTINGUISHING FEATURES
- Neovascularisation on the retina or optic disc
- Preretinal haemorrhage
- Tractional retinal detachment
- Neovascular glaucoma (new vessels on the iris and anterior chamber angle)

RED FLAGS
- Sudden floaters
- Sudden flashes of light
- Sudden loss of vision

Fig. 12.6 Proliferative diabetic retinopathy illness script (illness script 35)

Table 12.1 Comparison of diabetic maculopathy, non-proliferative and proliferative diabetic retinopathy illness scripts

	Diabetic maculopathy	Non-proliferative diabetic retinopathy	Proliferative diabetic retinopathy
Cause	Type 1 and 2 diabetes mellitus High sugar levels Leaky blood vessels Blocked blood vessels Swelling of the macula	Type 1 and 2 diabetes mellitus High sugar levels	Type 1 and 2 diabetes mellitus High sugar levels Hypoxia
Risk factors	Duration of diabetes Poor diabetic control Coexisting diseases (e.g. hypertension) Smoking Pregnancy	Diabetes duration Poor blood glucose control High blood pressure Dyslipidaemia Smoking Pregnancy	Duration of diabetes Younger age at diagnosis (especially type 1) Poor diabetic control Uncontrolled hypertension Dyslipidaemia Smoking Obesity Kidney disease Pregnancy Obstructive sleep apnoea Genetics and ethnicity: higher risk Asian, Afro-Caribbean, Latino descent Puberty

Mechanisms and pathogenesis	BRB breakdown: Leak out, fluid accumulation Closure of capillary network, non-perfusion (ischaemia), compensatory VEGF release Increased vascular permeability Inflammation, oxidative stress: damage cells and vascular injury Extracellular oedema Intracellular oedema Hard exudates Arteriovenous shunts	Vascular damage and permeability: Hyperglycaemia damages endothelial cells Microaneurysms form from weakened vessel walls, leaking blood and fluid Haemorrhages and exudates Ischaemia & inflammation Capillary occlusion Oxidative stress Inflammation VEGF signalling and vascular permeability	Chronic hyperglycaemia & ischemia: retinal blood vessels damage, leading to closure (non-perfusion), hypoxia VEGF stimulates neovascularization Bleed into the vitreous (vitreous haemorrhage) Fibrous scar tissue alongside new vessels Scar tissue contracts eventually causing a retinal detachment Oxidative stress, inflammation, glutamate excitotoxicity, microRNAs changes
Symptoms	Mild cases, vision can be normal Visual acuity gradual reduction Blurred or fluctuating central vision Distortion Colour vision and contrast loss Floaters, dark spots or shadows Photophobia	Often no early symptoms (vison normal) Blurred vision Floaters Scotomas Poor night vision Impaired colour vision	Vision can be normal Visual acuity may be reduced suddenly (vitreous haemorrhage) Floaters Flashing lights

(continued)

Table 12.1 (continued)

	Diabetic maculopathy	Non-proliferative diabetic retinopathy	Proliferative diabetic retinopathy
Signs	Microaneurysms Haemorrhages Exudates, circinate Retinal oedema Retinal ischaemia IRMAs	Venous beading and tortuosity, loops Arteriolar occlusions IRMA Microaneurysms Haemorrhages (dot and blot, flame-shaped), hard exudates (lipid deposits) Cotton wool spots (soft exudates)	In addition to signs of NPDR New vessels on the disc or retina elsewhere Neuroretina traction by fibrous proliferation
Complications	Diabetic macular oedema Ischemic maculopathy Retinal detachment Vitreous haemorrhage	Diabetic macular oedema Progression to proliferative diabetic retinopathy	Preretinal haemorrhage Vitreous haemorrhage Tractional retinal detachment Neovascular glaucoma
Natural history and prognosis	Severe vision loss/blindness, if complications like detachment or severe oedema not treated	Resolution/stabilization: some cases, especially in younger patients Progression to PDR can occur over years, rates vary but can be significant (e.g. 26–52% in 1 year for untreated severe NPDR) (IRMA risk factor of progression to PDR)	May progress despite treatment Potentially blinding Poor prognosis features: neovascularization on the optic disc or retina with haemorrhage Prognosis: with treatment (PRP +/− anti-VEGF injections) may maintain good vision (>6/12)

Investigations	General assessment Fundus examination OCT scan of the macula Fundus fluorescein angiography OCT angiography (assess retinal circulation non-invasively) Blood sugar Blood pressure control	General assessment Fundus examination OCT scan of the macula Fundus fluorescein angiography OCT angiography (assess retinal circulation non-invasively) Blood sugar Blood pressure control	General assessment Fundus examination OCT scan of the macula Fundus fluorescein angiography OCT angiography (assess retinal circulation non-invasively) Blood sugar Blood pressure control
Management	AntiVEGF Laser therapy aiming at points of leakage Intravitreal steroids Improve diabetes and cardiovascular control Avoid smoking	Retina laser Improve cardiovascular risk factors, underlying, hypertension, high cholesterol Avoid smoking	Scatter retinal laser photocoagulation (PRP) Intravitreal anti-VEGF injections Surgery (remove the vitreous gel/haemorrhage, repair and reattach the detached retina)

(continued)

Table 12.1 (continued)

	Diabetic maculopathy	Non-proliferative diabetic retinopathy	Proliferative diabetic retinopathy
Distinguishing features	Macular oedema Macular ischaemia Macular hard exudates Distorted, blurred central vision Dark spots in central vision Reduced contrast sensitivity Photophobia	Peripheral retina Intraretinal microvascular abnormalities Microaneurysms Haemorrhages (e.g. dot-blot, deeper layers) Hard exudates Cotton wool spots Venous beading, dilation Absence of neovascularization	Neovascularization on the retina or optic disc Vitreous or preretinal haemorrhage Tractional retinal detachment Neovascular glaucoma (new vessels on the iris and anterior chamber angle)
Red flags	Worsening central vision (blurred, distortion) Dark spots/floaters/smudges central vision Faded colours, difficulty with fine details Sudden vision loss	Floaters/spots Blurred/cloudy vision Dark or empty spots Difficulty in low light Faded colours	Sudden floaters/cobwebs Sudden vision loss, darkness Poor night vision Flashes of light Faded colours, washed out

Hypertensive Retinopathy 13

Hypertensive retinopathy is categorized into different grades, with distinct features: (a) mild chronic retinopathy, chronic vascular changes develop over a long period of elevated blood pressure, (b) moderate acute retinopathy, with vascular changes related to a combination of high blood pressure, vascular leakage and ischaemia and (c) severe malignant retinopathy, a sign of a hypertensive crisis and a medical emergency. One of the hallmarks of severe hypertensive retinopathy is optic disc swelling. It indicates potential end-organ damage (e.g. brain and kidneys) (Figs. 13.1, 13.2, 13.3, 13.4, 13.5, and 13.6).

The following illness scripts (Figs. 13.2, 13.4, and 13.6) and Table 13.1 compare the elements mild chronic, moderate acute and malignant hypertensive retinopathy.

M. Ugarte, *Ophthalmology Illness Scripts*,
https://doi.org/10.1007/978-3-032-31008-8_13

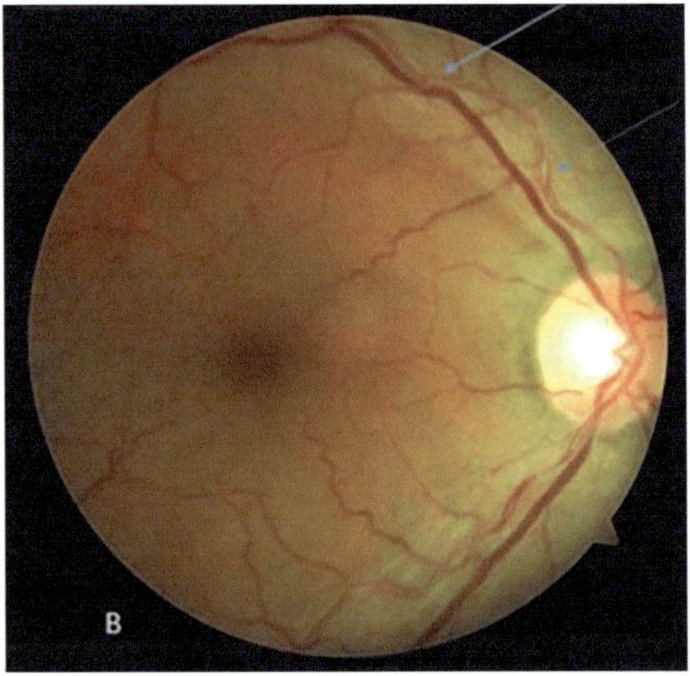

SIGNS

- Arterial narrowing (white arrow)
- Arterio-venous (AV) nicking (nipping) (black arrow) (arteries pressing on veins)
- Arterial "silver and copper wiring" (thickened artery walls) (arrow)

Fig. 13.1 Mild chronic hypertensive retinopathy

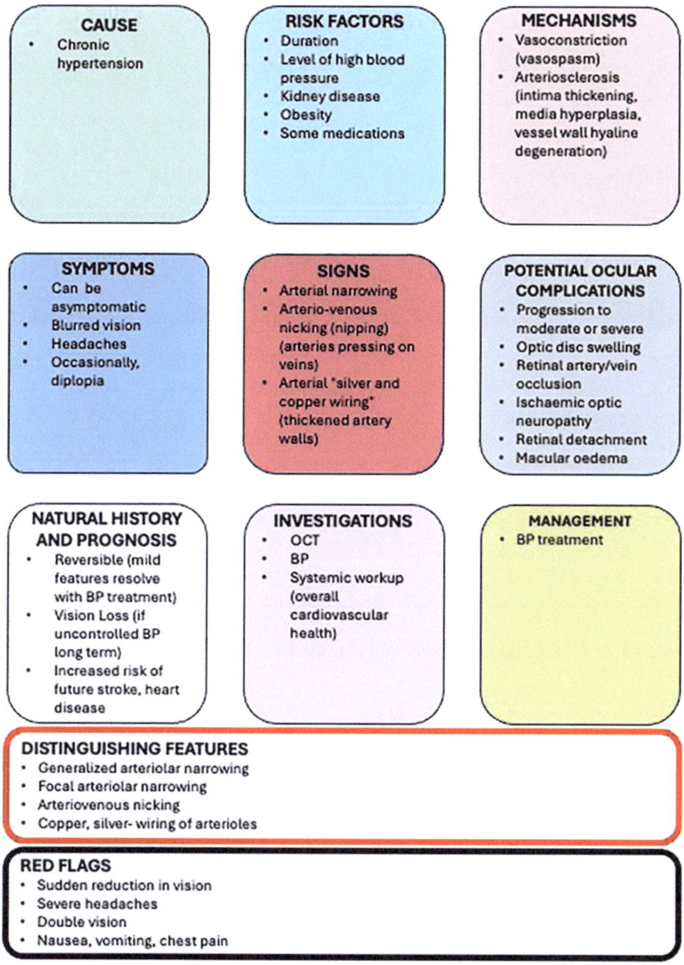

Fig. 13.2 Mild chronic hypertensive retinopathy illness script (illness script 36)

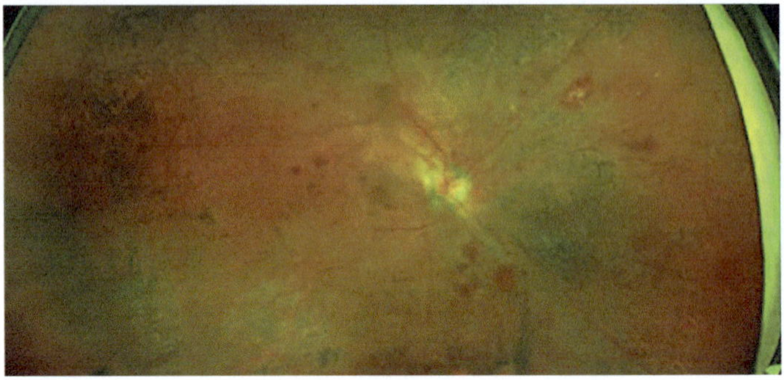

SIGNS

- Arterial narrowing
- AV nicking
- Arterial "silver and copper wiring"
- Retinal haemorrhages
- Hard exudates
- Cotton-wool spots

Fig. 13.3 Moderate hypertensive retinopathy

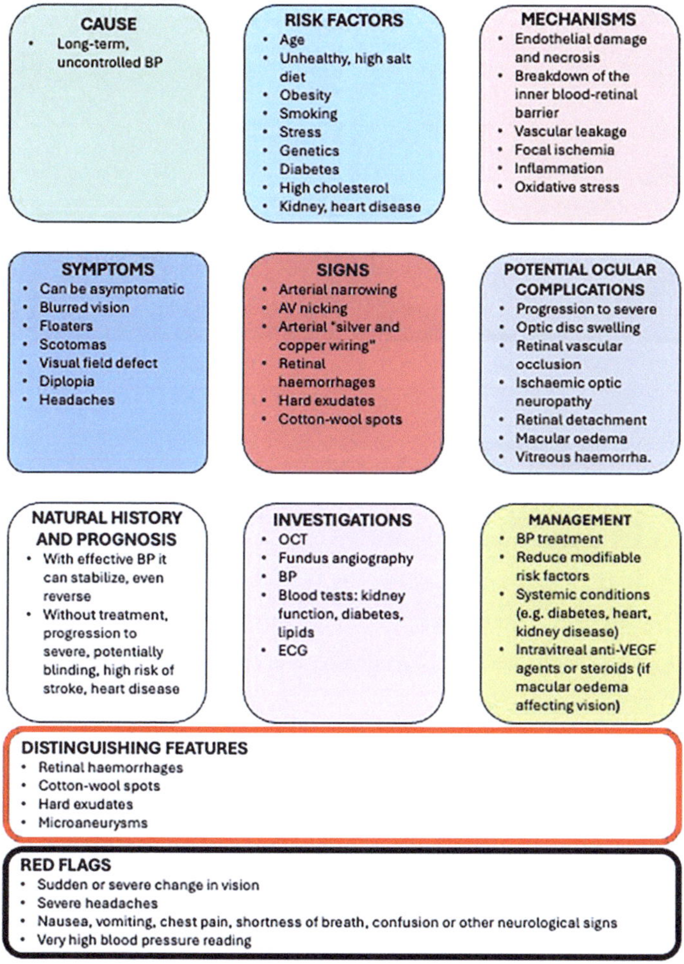

Fig. 13.4 Moderate acute hypertensive retinopathy illness script (illness script 37)

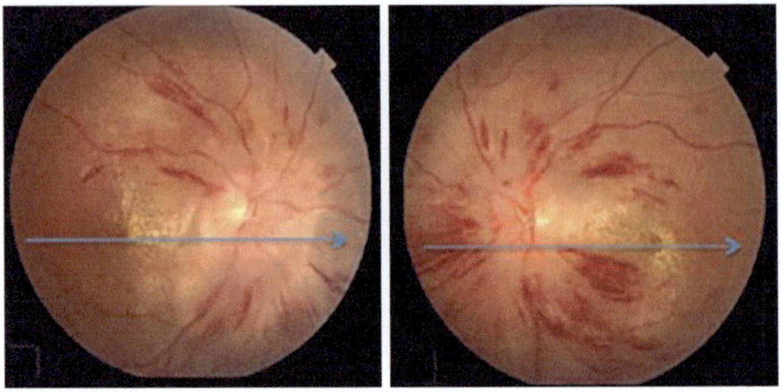

SIGNS

- Arterial narrowing
- AV nicking
- Arterial "silver and copper wiring"
- Retinal haemorrhages
- Hard exudates
- Cotton-wool spots
- Swollen optic disc

Fig. 13.5 Severe malignant hypertensive retinopathy

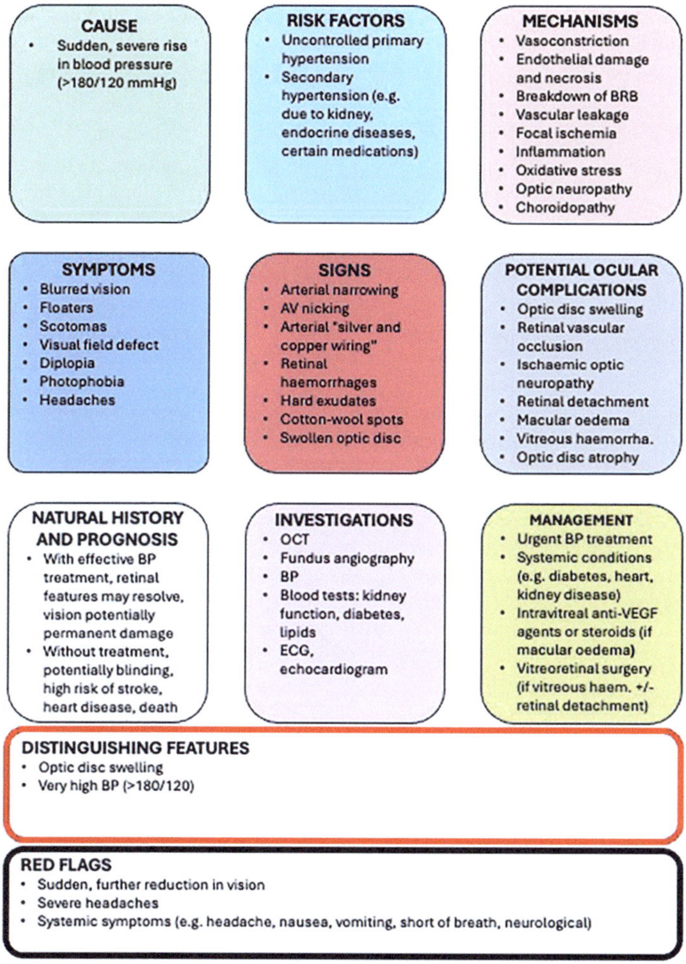

Fig. 13.6 Severe malignant hypertensive retinopathy illness script (illness script 38)

Table 13.1 Comparison of mild chronic, moderate acute and severe malignant hypertensive retinopathy illness scripts

	Mild chronic hypertensive retinopathy	Moderate acute hypertensive retinopathy	Severe malignant hypertensive retinopathy
Cause	Chronic hypertension	Long-term, uncontrolled BP	Sudden, severe rise in blood pressure (>180/120 mmHg)
Risk factors	Duration Level of high blood pressure Kidney disease Obesity Some medications	Age Unhealthy, high salt diet Obesity Smoking Stress Genetics Diabetes High cholesterol Kidney, heart disease	Uncontrolled primary hypertension Secondary hypertension (e.g. due to kidney, endocrine diseases, certain medications)
Mechanisms and pathogenesis	Vasoconstriction (vasospasm) Arteriosclerosis (intima thickening, media hyperplasia, vessel wall hyaline degeneration)	Endothelial damage and necrosis Breakdown of the inner blood-retinal barrier Vascular leakage Focal ischemia Inflammation Oxidative stress	Vasoconstriction Endothelial damage and necrosis Breakdown of BRB Vascular leakage Focal ischemia Inflammation Oxidative stress Optic neuropathy Choroidopathy
Symptoms	Can be asymptomatic Blurred vision Headaches Occasionally, diplopia	Can be asymptomatic Blurred vision Floaters Scotomas Visual field defect Diplopia Headaches	Blurred vision Floaters Scotomas Visual field defect Diplopia Photophobia Headaches

(continued)

Table 13.1 (continued)

	Mild chronic hypertensive retinopathy	Moderate acute hypertensive retinopathy	Severe malignant hypertensive retinopathy
Signs	Arterial narrowing Arterio-venous nicking (nipping) (arteries pressing on veins) Arterial "silver and copper wiring" (thickened artery walls)	Arterial narrowing AV nicking Arterial "silver and copper wiring" Retinal haemorrhages Hard exudates Cotton-wool spots	Arterial narrowing AV nicking Arterial "silver and copper wiring" Retinal haemorrhages Hard exudates Cotton-wool spots Swollen optic disc
Complications	Progression to moderate or severe Optic disc swelling Retinal artery/vein occlusion Ischaemic optic neuropathy Retinal detachment Macular oedema	Progression to severe Optic disc swelling Retinal vascular occlusion Ischaemic optic neuropathy Retinal detachment Macular oedema Vitreous haemorrhage	Optic disc swelling Retinal vascular occlusion Ischaemic optic neuropathy Retinal detachment Macular oedema Vitreous haemorrhage Optic disc atrophy
Natural history and prognosis	Reversible (mild features resolve with BP treatment) Vision loss (if uncontrolled BP long term) Increased risk of future stroke, heart disease	With effective BP it can stabilize, even reverse Without treatment, progression to severe, potentially blinding, high risk of stroke, heart disease	With effective BP treatment, retinal features may resolve, vision potentially permanent damage Without treatment, potentially blinding, high risk of stroke, heart disease, death

(continued)

Table 13.1 (continued)

	Mild chronic hypertensive retinopathy	Moderate acute hypertensive retinopathy	Severe malignant hypertensive retinopathy
Investigations	OCT BP Systemic workup (overall cardiovascular health)	OCT Fundus angiography BP Blood tests: kidney function, diabetes, lipids ECG	OCT Fundus angiography BP Blood tests: kidney function, diabetes, lipids ECG, echocardiogram
Management	BP treatment	BP treatment Reduce modifiable risk factors Systemic conditions (e.g. diabetes, heart, kidney disease) Intravitreal anti-VEGF agents or steroids (if macular oedema affecting vision)	Urgent BP treatment Systemic conditions (e.g. diabetes, heart, kidney disease) Intravitreal anti-VEGF agents or steroids (if macular oedema) Vitreoretinal surgery (if vitreous haem. +/– retinal detachment)
Distinguishing features	Generalized arteriolar narrowing Focal arteriolar narrowing Arteriovenous nicking Copper, silver-wiring of arterioles	Retinal haemorrhages Cotton-wool spots Hard exudates Microaneurysms	Optic disc swelling Very high BP (>180/120)

(continued)

Table 13.1 (continued)

	Mild chronic hypertensive retinopathy	Moderate acute hypertensive retinopathy	Severe malignant hypertensive retinopathy
Red flags	Sudden reduction in vision Severe headaches Double vision Nausea, vomiting, chest pain	Sudden or severe change in vision Severe headaches Nausea, vomiting, chest pain, shortness of breath, confusion or other neurological signs Very high blood pressure reading	Sudden, further reduction in vision Severe headaches Systemic symptoms (e.g. headache, nausea, vomiting, short of breath, neurological symptoms)

Age-Related Macular Degeneration and Inherited Macular Dystrophy

14

Age-related macular degeneration is classified into two groups: non-exudative (dry) (Figs. 14.1 and 14.2) and exudative (wet) (Figs. 14.3 and 14.4), which are primarily distinguished by the absence or presence of abnormal growing blood vessels in the choroid and underneath the retina (i.e. choroidal neovascularization or macular vascular network), respectively. Inherited macular dystrophies (Figs. 14.5 and 14.6) include a group of conditions with specific types, different age onsets, rate of progression and/or retinal features (e.g. Stargardt disease, Sorsby fundus dystrophy, pattern dystrophy, cone-rod dystrophy).

The following illness scripts (Figs. 14.2, 14.4, and 14.6) and Table 14.1 describe and compare the elements of non-exudative and exudative age-related macular degeneration and inherited macular dystrophy.

M. Ugarte, *Ophthalmology Illness Scripts*,
https://doi.org/10.1007/978-3-032-31008-8_14

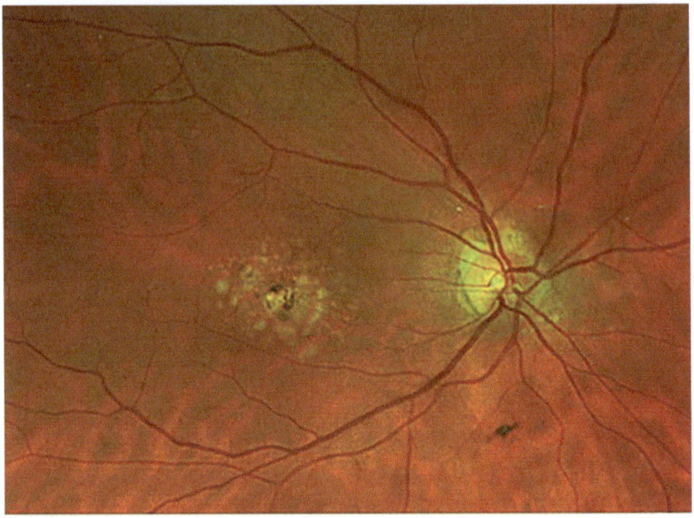

SIGNS

- Drusen (yellow deposits) in the macula
- Hypo and hyperpigmentation
- Areas of retina atrophy

Fig. 14.1 Non-exudative age-related macular degeneration

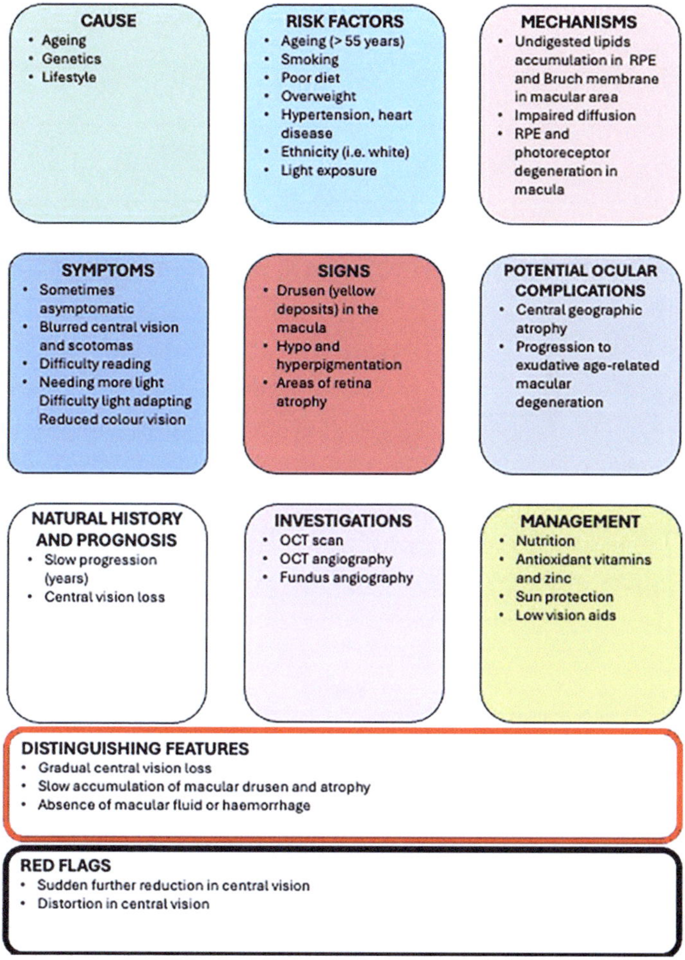

Fig. 14.2 Non-exudative age-related macular degeneration illness script (illness script 39)

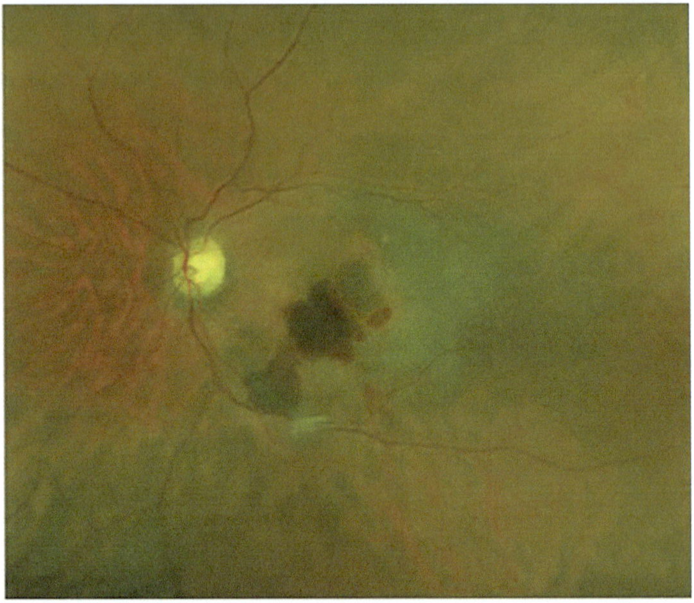

SIGNS

- Large or confluent macular drusen
- Fluid exudation +/ blood in the subretinal space or within the retina
- Hypo- and hyperpigmentation
- Arass of atrophy

Fig. 14.3 Exudative age-related macular degeneration

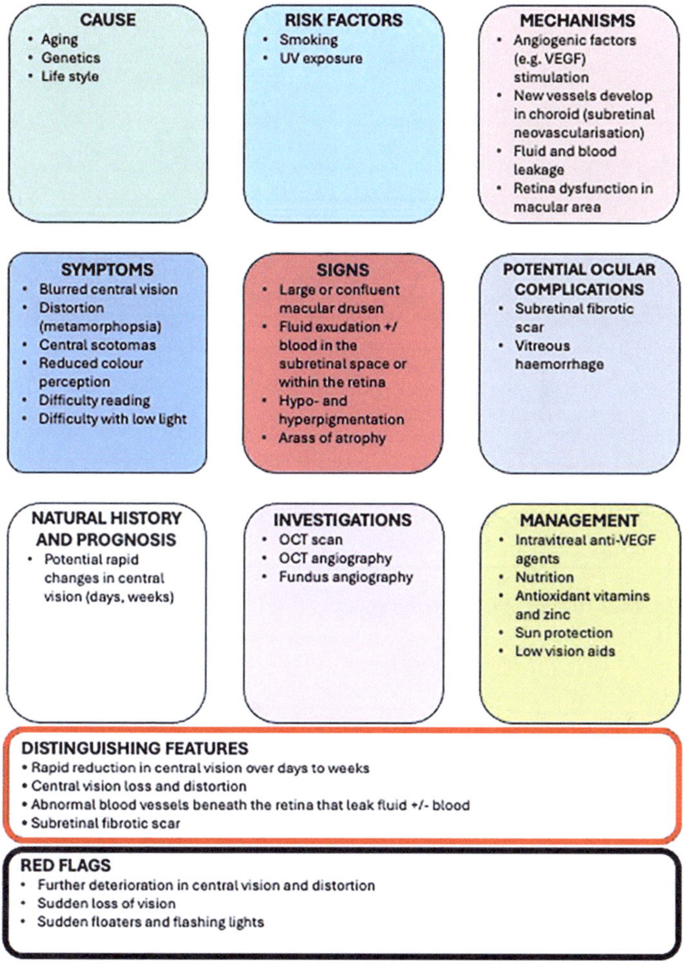

Fig. 14.4 Exudative age-related macular degeneration illness script (illness script 40)

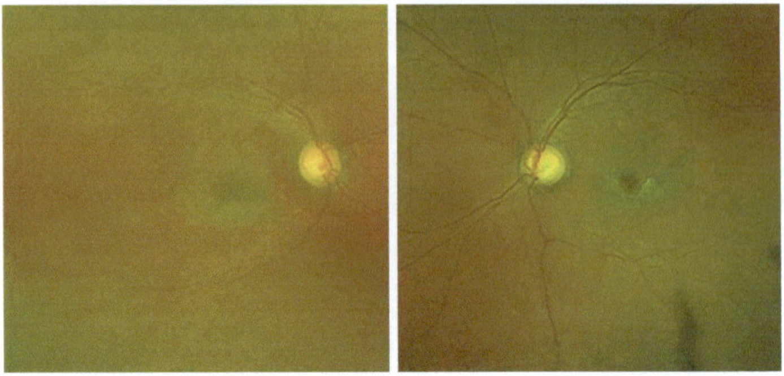

SIGNS

- Macula pigment changes
- +/- flecks and deposits
- +/- drusen
- +/- areas of atrophy
- +/- vascular changes
- +/- choroidal neovascularisation

Fig. 14.5 Inherited macular dystrophy

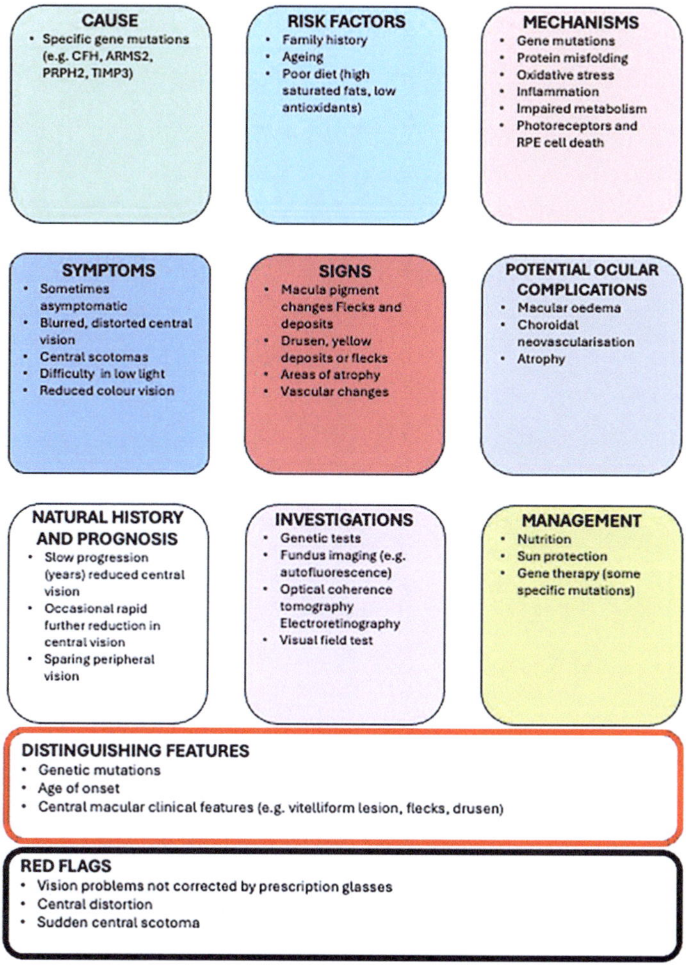

Fig. 14.6 Inherited macular dystrophy illness script (illness script 41)

Table 14.1 Comparison of non-exudative and exudative age-related macular degeneration and inherited macular dystrophy illness scripts

	Non-exudative age-related macular degeneration	Exudative age-related macular degeneration	Inherited macular dystrophy
Cause	Ageing Genetics Lifestyle	Ageing Genetics Life style	Specific gene mutations (like in *CFH*, *ARMS2*, PRPH2, TIMP3)
Risk factors	Ageing (increasing after age 50) Genetics (complement factor H) Smoking Diet (high saturated fats, low leafy greens/omega-3s) Overweight, hypertension, heart disease Race (white) Light exposure	Smoking UV exposure	Family history Modifiable factors Smoking Age Poor diet (high saturated fats, low antioxidants) Obesity, hypertension Northern European descent

Mechanisms and pathogensis	Undigested lipid products (e.g. age pigment lipofuscin) accumulate in the RPE and the excess material is transferred to Bruch membrane, impairing its diffusional properties The neighbouring RPE and photoreceptors show degenerative changes Does not spread to affect the peripheral vision Tissue degeneration	New vessels from the choroid Subretinal neovascular membrane stimulated by angiogenic factors (e.g. VEGF) grow through defects in Bruch membrane and RPE into SRS Detached neuroretina from the RPE Leakage of fluid and blood Disruption of macular function Rapid central vision loss	Gene mutations Protein misfolding Oxidative stress Inflammation Impaired metabolism Cell death, structural breakdown Disrupt macula cell function, primarily photoreceptors and RPE Progressive damage Vision loss

(continued)

Table 14.1 (continued)

	Non-exudative age-related macular degeneration	Exudative age-related macular degeneration	Inherited macular dystrophy
Symptoms	Vision can be normal Blurred central vision Words disappearing when reading Needing more light for close work Difficulty adapting to low light Reduced colour perception Distortion Micropsia, macropsia Scotomas Navigational vision is retained Symptoms mild or absent in early stages	Blurred central vision Reduced colour perception Distortion, wavy lines (metamorphopsia): Micropsia, macropsia Central scotomas Difficulty seeing in low light Difficulty reading, driving, or recognizing faces Straight lines wavy, distorted Blind spots in central vision	Specific patterns of vision loss Night blindness Difficulty seeing in low light Reduced colour vision Blurred or distorted central vision Dark spots, reading, facial recognition Wavy/bent straight lines Family history of the condition Family history of vision loss though peripheral vision usually intact longer Severity and onset vary by type

Signs	Early AMD: Drusen (yellow deposits) RPE hypo and hyperpigmentation Advanced AMD: geographic atrophy Large or confluent drusen Hypo- and hyperpigmentation	Fluid exudation into the sub-retinal space or into the retina SubRPE, subretinal, preretinal haemorrhage Large or confluent drusen Hypo- and hyperpigmentation Atrophy	Pigment changes atrophy in macula Flecks and deposits Drusen, yellow deposits Atrophy Vascular changes
Complications	Central geographic atrophy (GA)	Subretinal fibrotic scar Vitreous haemorrhage	Macular oedema Cataract Choroidal neovascularisation Atrophy
Natural history and pathogenesis	Progresses slowly over years Years asymptomatic Drusen enlargement Atrophy of RPE and photoreceptors GA often starting peripherally, hits the fovea	Rapid changes in vision over a relatively short period	Progressive macular atrophy Ultimately affecting central sight but often sparing peripheral vision

(continued)

Table 14.1 (continued)

	Non-exudative age-related macular degeneration	Exudative age-related macular degeneration	Inherited macular dystrophy
Investigations	Fundal exam Macula OCT scan OCT angiography Fundus fluorescein angiography, indocyanine green angiography (ICG)	Fundal exam Optical coherence tomography OCT OCT angiography Fundus fluorescein angiography, ICG	Genetic testing, definitive diagnosis Fundus autofluorescence Optical coherence tomography Electroretinograms Visual fields
Management	Antioxidant vitamins and zinc Nutrition Sun protection Low vision aids	Intravitreal anti-VEGF Low visual aid	Gene therapy Nutrition
Distinguishing features	Minimal or no early symptoms Gradual central vision loss Slow accumulation of drusen Gradual retinal pigment epithelium atrophy Absence of fluid or haemorrhage	Rapid onset over days to weeks Central vision loss or distortion Abnormal blood vessels beneath the retina that leak fluid or blood (PED, SRF, IRF) Disciform scar	Specific clinical signs Genetic tests Age of onset
Red flags	Distortion in central vision	Wavy or distorted straight lines Dark or blurry spot in your central vision	Vision problems not corrected by prescription glasses Central distortion Sudden central scotoma

15 Retinal Detachment

Retinal detachment is a serious eye condition where the neuroretina separates from the retina pigment epithelium, potentially causing permanent vision loss, and requires urgent medical attention. Symptoms include new floaters, flashes of light, blurred vision or a shadow/curtain in the field of vision. It often happens when the vitreous gel pulls on the retina, creating a tear that lets fluid seep underneath, but can also be caused by inflammation or diabetic eye disease. Treatment depends on the type (rhegmatogenous, tractional, exudative) (Figs. 15.1, 15.2, 15.3, 15.4, 15.5, and 15.6).

The distinguishing features of a retinal detachment are their key symptoms and clinical signs observed during an eye exam. The following illness scripts (Figs. 15.2, 15.4, and 15.6) and Table 15.1 compare the elements rhegmatogenous, serous and tractional retinal detachment, highlighting the specific distinguishing features and red flags.

M. Ugarte, *Ophthalmology Illness Scripts*,
https://doi.org/10.1007/978-3-032-31008-8_15

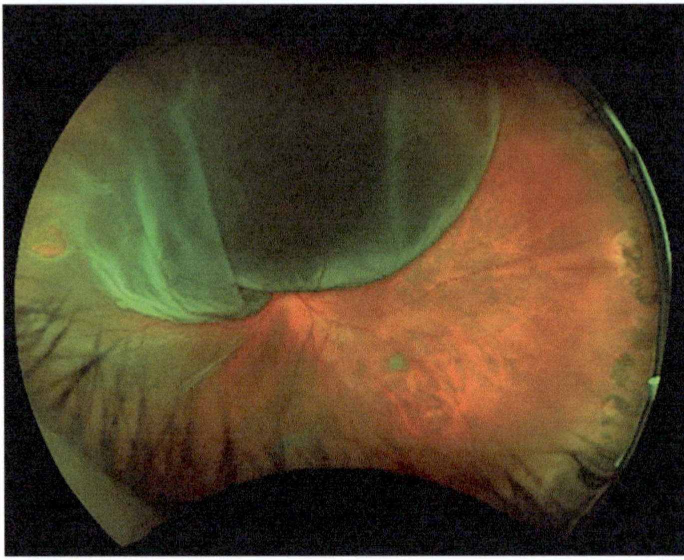

SIGNS

- Fluid in the subretinal space
- Floating, corrugated retina, undulating with eye movements
- Break in the retina
- Debris in the vitreous (e.g. blood, pigment)

Fig. 15.1 Rhegmatogenous retinal detachment

CAUSE
- Retinal break (i.e. tear or hole)

RISK FACTORS
- Posterior vitreous detachment
- Peripheral retinal lattice degeneration
- High myopia
- Cataract surgery
- Previous detached retina in fellow eye
- Trauma
- Family history of retinal detachment

MECHANISMS
- Liquefied vitreous gains entry to the subretinal space via a retinal break
- Neuroretina separates from the RPE

SYMPTOMS
- Usually sudden
- Painless
- Visual field defect ('shadow' or 'curtain')
- Increased floaters
- Flashes of light
- Central vision reduction (if macula detached)

SIGNS
- Fluid in the subretinal space
- Floating, corrugated retina, undulating with eye movements
- Break in the retina
- Debris in the vitreous (e.g. blood, pigment)

POTENTIAL OCULAR COMPLICATIONS
- Complete, permanent vision loss
- Intraocular inflammation
- Retina ischaemia
- Strabismus
- Retina +/- iris neovascularisation

NATURAL HISTORY AND PROGNOSIS
- Rapid progression (hours, days)
- Surgical reattachment good prognosis
- Potential recurrence

INVESTIGATIONS
- Optical coherence tomography (OCT) (determine if macula attached or detached)
- Ultrasound B-Scan (if poor fundal view)

MANAGEMENT
- Vitreoretinal surgery

DISTINGUISHING FEATURES
- Rapid onset of symptoms
- Corrugated, undulating retina
- Subretinal fluid (non shifting)
- Retinal break

RED FLAGS
- Sudden floaters
- Sudden flashes of light
- Sudden shadow, visual field defect
- Progression of central vision loss

Fig. 15.2 Rhegmatogenous retinal detachment illness script (illness script 42)

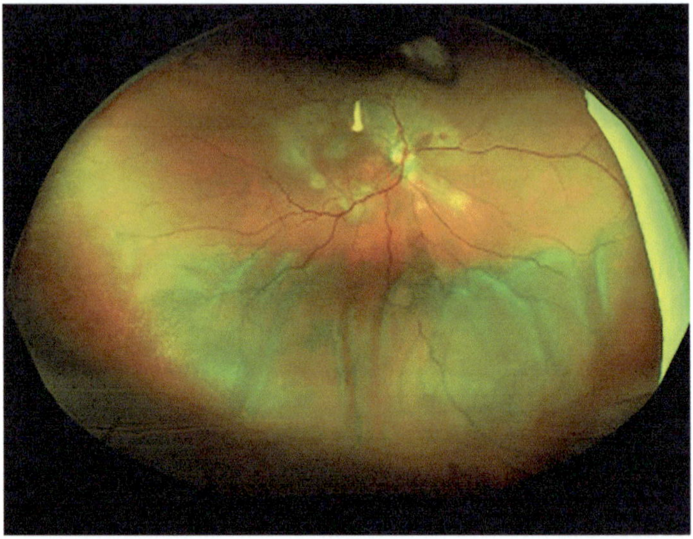

SIGNS

- Subretinal fluid (shifts with head position, gravity-dependent)
- Convex, smooth retinal surface

Fig. 15.3 Exudative retinal detachment

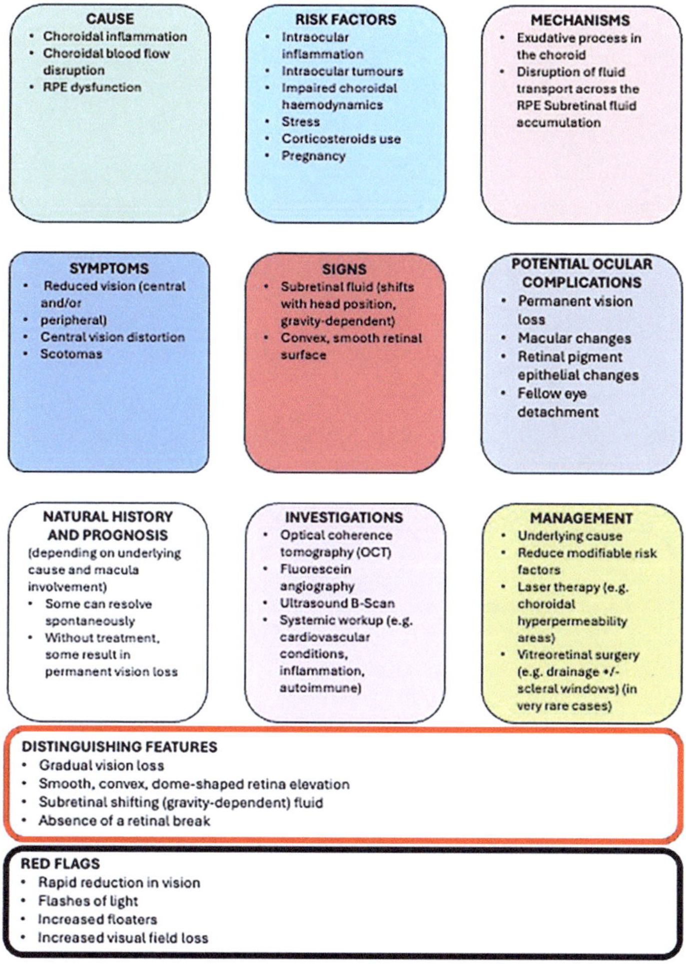

Fig. 15.4 Serous retinal detachment illness script (illness script 43)

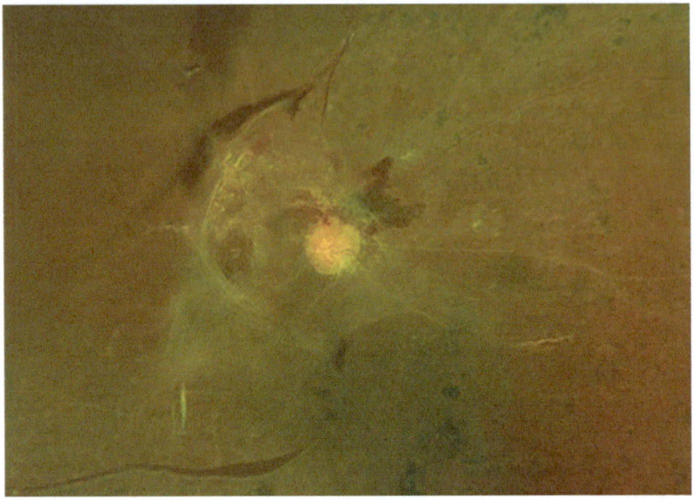

SIGNS

- Concave retina elevation
- Preretinal fibrotic tissue
- Absence of retinal mobility
- Absence of retinal breaks

Fig. 15.5 Tractional retinal detachment

CAUSE
- Contracting fibrous tissue on the retinal surface

RISK FACTORS
- Proliferative retinopathy (e.g. PDR)
- Trauma
- Previous retina surgery
- Intraocular inflammation

MECHANISMS
- Contraction of fibrovascular tissue on retina inner surface
- Mechanical traction
- Neuroretina pulled away from the RPE

SYMPTOMS
- Gradual loss of vision
- Distortion
- Visual field defect

SIGNS
- Concave retina elevation
- Preretinal fibrotic tissue
- Absence of retinal mobility
- Absence of retinal breaks

POTENTIAL OCULAR COMPLICATIONS
- Permanent vision loss
- Retinal ischaemia
- Vitreous haemorrhage
- Retina break
- Combined rhegmatogenous retinal detachment
- Neovascular glaucoma

NATURAL HISTORY AND PROGNOSIS
- Untreated, often severe, permanent vision loss
- Following vitreoretinal surgery, good prognosis
- Recurrence
- Potentially blinding

INVESTIGATIONS
- Optical coherence tomography (OCT)
- Fluorescein angiography
- Ultrasound B-Scan

MANAGEMENT
- Observation (if no progression)
- Vitreoretinal surgery

DISTINGUISHING FEATURES
- Preretinal fibrous tissue
- Concave, immobile retina elevation
- Shallow subretinal fluid, non-shifting
- Absence of retinal break

RED FLAGS
- Sudden increased floaters
- Sudden increased flashes of light
- Rapid progression of shadow, visual field defect
- Rapid further reduction in vision

Fig. 15.6 Tractional retinal detachment illness script (illness script 44)

Table 15.1 Comparison of rhegmatogenous, serous and tractional retinal detachment illness scripts

	Rhegmatogenous retinal detachment	Serous retinal detachment	Tractional retinal detachment
Cause	Retinal break (tear or hole)	Choroidal inflammation Choroidal blood flow disruption RPE dysfunction	Contracting fibrous tissue on the retinal surface, which pulls off the neuroretina
Risk factors	Posterior vitreous detachment Peripheral retinal lattice degeneration High myopia Previous cataract surgery (if complicated) Previous detached retina in fellow Trauma Family history of retinal detachment	Intraocular inflammation Tumours Impaired choroidal blood flow, haemodynamics, high blood pressure, corticosteroids, pregnancy	Proliferative retinopathy (e.g. PDR) Trauma Previous retina surgery Intraocular inflammation
Mechanisms and pathogenesis	Liquefied vitreous gains entry to the subretinal space via a retinal break Neuroretina separates from the RPE	Exudative process in the choroid and/or disruption of fluid transport across the RPE Fluid accumulates in the sub-retinal space	Fibrovascular tissue on retina inner surface Contraction, mechanical traction Neuroretina pulled away from the RPE

(continued)

Table 15.1 (continued)

	Rhegmatogenous retinal detachment	Serous retinal detachment	Tractional retinal detachment
Symptoms	Typically sudden Painless Visual field defect (“shadow” or “curtain”) Increased floaters Flashes of light (photopsia) progressing centrally Central severe reduction (macula detached)	Central vision Peripheral vision Distortion Scotoma Blurring Distortion Blind spots	Gradual loss of vision Blurring Distortion Curtain
Signs	Fluid in the sub-retinal space Floating, diaphanous membrane Undulating retina with eye movements Corrugated retinal appearance Break in the retina Debris in the vitreous (e.g. blood, pigment)	Subretinal fluid shifts with head position, gravity-dependent Convex, smooth retinal surface Absence of a retinal tear	Concave retinal configuration Impaired retinal mobility Fibrotic tissue Absence of retinal breaks
Complications	Complete permanent vision loss: Intraocular inflammation Ischaemia Strabismus	Permanent vision loss Macular changes Retinal pigment epithelial changes Fellow eye detachment	Vision loss Retinal ischaemia Vitreous haemorrhage Neovascular glaucoma Proliferative Vitreoretinopathy, scar tissue

(continued)

Table 15.1 (continued)

	Rhegmatogenous retinal detachment	Serous retinal detachment	Tractional retinal detachment
Natural history and prognosis	Progression rapid over hours or days If surgery successfully reattaches the peripheral retina and the macula is attached, the outlook for vision is excellent If the macula is detached for more than 24 h prior to surgery, the previous visual acuity will not recover completely If the retina not successfully attached, surgery is complicated, fibrotic changes may occur and cause traction recurrence Outlook for vision is poor	Vary significantly depending on the underlying cause and macula involvement Without treatment, permanent vision loss is a high risk Central serous chorioretinopathy can resolve spontaneously	Untreated, often severe vision loss or blindness Vitrectomy offers good outcomes, especially if the macula is still attached, with high reattachment rates Complex cases or chronic detachment (macula off) worse visual recovery Recurrence

(continued)

Table 15.1 (continued)

	Rhegmatogenous retinal detachment	Serous retinal detachment	Tractional retinal detachment
Investigations	Optical coherence tomography Fundus fluorescein angiography Ultrasound B-Scan: Used if the view is obscured (e.g. dense cataract, haemorrhage) to locate the detachment	Optical coherence tomography Fundus fluorescein angiography B-Scan ultrasound Systemic workup: Since SRD often stems from RPE dysfunction due to systemic issues (e.g. inflammation)	Optical coherence tomography Fundus fluorescein angiography Ocular ultrasound
Management	Surgical techniques for repairing a retinal detachment 1. External (conventional approach) 2. Internal (vitreoretinal surgery) This relieves the vitreous traction on the retinal hole and apposes the RPE to the neuroretina	Treating underlying causes Medical management Corticosteroids Anti-VEGF agents Laser therapy (photocoagulation) Drainage Scleral window surgery	Vitreoretinal surgery, requiring excision of the contracting bands Vitrectomy Membrane peeling/dissection Tamponade Laser photocoagulation:

(continued)

Table 15.1 (continued)

	Rhegmatogenous retinal detachment	Serous retinal detachment	Tractional retinal detachment
Distinguishing features	Rapid onset Retinal break Corrugated, undulating retina Subretinal fluid (non-shifting) Lower intraocular pressure The presence of pigment granules in the anterior vitreous	Gradually progressive vision loss Smooth, convex, dome-shaped elevation Subretinal fluid accumulation, which shifts with changes in body position Absence of a retinal tear Potential underlying causes such as inflammation, tumours, or systemic conditions high blood pressure, corticosteroids, pregnancy	Gradually progressive vision loss, distortion Fibrous tissue, NVE, NVD Concave, immobile retina Shallow SRF, non-shifting Underlying condition (e.g. PDR)
Red flags	Sudden floaters Flashes of light (photopsia) Shadow/curtain: A grey or dark shadow appearing in your side vision (periphery) gradually spreading Progression of central vision loss	Flashes of light (photopsia) Floaters Field loss Failing vision	Sudden floaters Flashes of light (photopsias) Shadow/curtain Blurred or distorted vision Persistent blurriness or wavy vision Sudden vision loss

16 Optic Neuritis and Optic Neuropathy

Optic neuritis involves inflammation (often linked to demyelination) causing painful, rapid vision loss, colour desaturation, and usually disc swelling, typically in younger adults. Optic neuropathy is broader nerve damage/degeneration, often painless, onset of symptoms can be sudden or gradual, affecting colour/vision, with potential causes like ischemia (e.g. arteritic and non-arteritic anterior ischaemic optic neuropathy), toxins or inherited conditions (e.g. Leber's hereditary optic neuropathy). Distinguishing features include the presence or absence of pain, onset of symptoms and optic disc appearance (Figs. 16.1, 16.2, 16.3, 16.4, 16.5, and 16.6).

The following illness scripts (Figs. 16.2, 16.4, and 16.6) and Table 16.1 compare the elements of optic neuritis, ischaemic optic neuropathy and Leber's hereditary optic neuropathy.

M. Ugarte, *Ophthalmology Illness Scripts*,
https://doi.org/10.1007/978-3-032-31008-8_16

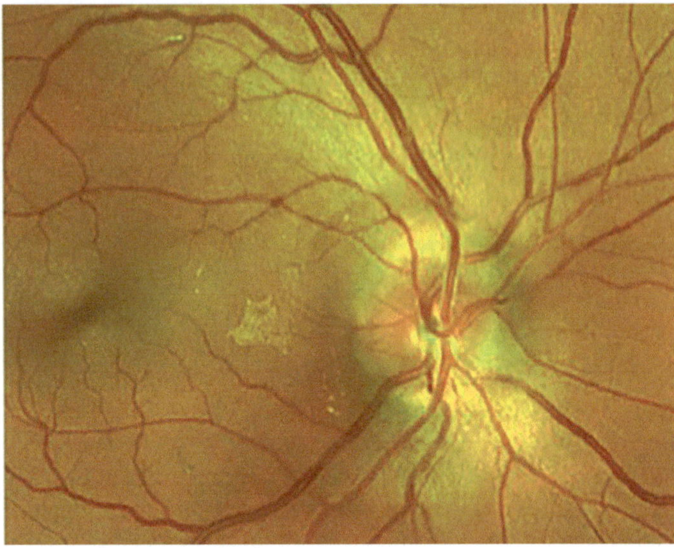

SIGNS

- Relative afferent pupillary defect
- Optic disc appearance: might be normal or swollen

Fig. 16.1 Optic neuritis

CAUSE
- Inflammation
- Autoimmune (e.g. MS, NMO)
- Infections (e.g. mumps, Lyme disease, syphilis)

RISK FACTORS
- Female
- Age 20-40 years
- White ethnicity
- Autoimmune disease
- Northern hemisphere
- Previous viral Infections

MECHANISMS
- Autoimmune response
- Inflammation
- Trigger: viral infection, MS or NMO
- Demyelination
- Nerve conduction block
- Axonal damage

SYMPTOMS
- Sudden vision loss
- Reduced colour vision (especially red)
- Visual field loss (central or peripheral)
- Flashing lights
- Heat-induced worsening
- Often 1 eye (might be bilateral sequential)
- Pain (behind eye) worse with movement

SIGNS
- Relative afferent pupillary defect
- Optic disc appearance: might be normal or swollen

POTENTIAL OCULAR COMPLICATIONS
- Optic atrophy

NATURAL HISTORY AND PROGNOSIS
- Sudden onset
- Worsen over hours-days
- Self-recovery over weeks to months (most close to normal)
- Recurrence (approximately 50% of MS-related optic neuritis within 5 years)

INVESTIGATIONS
- MRI head and orbit
- Blood tests (for aquaporin 4, MGO antibodies, exclude infections, autoimmune conditions)
- Visual evoked potential
- Lumbar puncture

MANAGEMENT
- Referral to ophthalmology and/or neurology
- Observation (may improve spontaneously)
- Systemic steroids
- Plasma exchange
- Immunosuppressants (in certain cases)

DISTINGUISHING FEATURES
- Age at presentation
- Pain on eye movement
- Spontaneous recovery
- Optic nerve inflammation seen on MRI a

RED FLAGS
- Bilateral simultaneously or sequential involvement
- Severe vision loss
- Painless onset
- Poor steroid response

Fig. 16.2 Optic neuritis illness script (illness script 45)

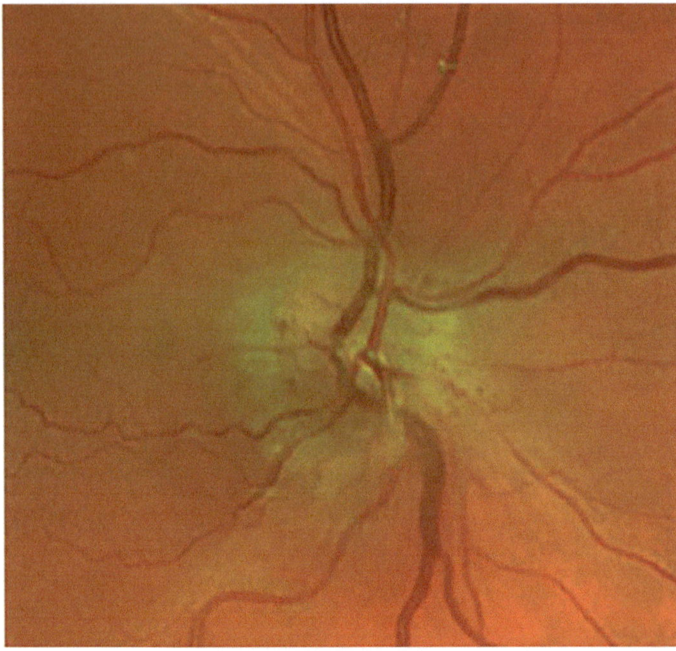

SIGNS

- Optic disc appearance: swollen, chalky white, haemorrhages
- Visual field defect (usually altitudinal)
- •Relative afferent pupillary defect

Fig. 16.3 Anterior ischemic optic neuropathy

CAUSE
- Ischaemia

RISK FACTORS
- Age (>50 years)
- Diabetes
- Hypertension
- Hypercholesterolaemia
- Smoking
- Obstructive sleep apnoea
- Giant cell arteritis (i.e. arteritic type)

MECHANISMS
- Reduced optic nerve posterior ciliary arteries blood supply
- Ischaemia
- Excitotoxicity
- Oxidative stress
- Apoptosis
- Retinal ganglion cell death
- Axonal degeneration

SYMPTOMS
- Sudden vision loss
- Visual field defect (usually altitudinal)
- Reduced colour vision (washed out)
- Some cases eye pain
- Some cases systemic symptoms of GCA (i.e. arteritic type)

SIGNS
- Visual field defect (usually altitudinal)
- •Relative afferent pupillary defect
- Optic disc appearance: swollen, chalky white, haemorrhages

POTENTIAL OCULAR COMPLICATIONS
- Optic disc atrophy
- Fellow eye affected

NATURAL HISTORY AND PROGNOSIS
- Sudden onset
- Occasional recovery(up to 40% non-arteritic type)
- •Permanent visual loss
- •Fellow eye affected (e.g. without treatment in arteritic type)
- Recurrence

INVESTIGATIONS
- BP
- Blood Tests: cardiovascular risk factors, ESR. CRP
- MRI head and orbits (if suspected CNS pathology, compression)

MANAGEMENT
- Urgent systemic sterois treatment in arteritic type,
- Optimise cardiovascular risk factors
- Low vision aids

DISTINGUISHING FEATURES
- Age at presentation
- Arteritic type: elevated inflammatory markers (ESR, CRP), associated GCA symptoms
- Non arteritic type: cardiovascular risk factors, normal inflammatory markers, no associated symptoms of GCA

RED FLAGS
- GCA signs and/or symptoms (scalp tenderness, jaw claudication, pain, fatigue, PMR, general malaise)
- History of amaurosis fugax
- Rapidly sequential bilateral vision loss
- Elevated inflammatory markers.

Fig. 16.4 Anterior ischaemic optic neuropathy illness script (illness script 46)

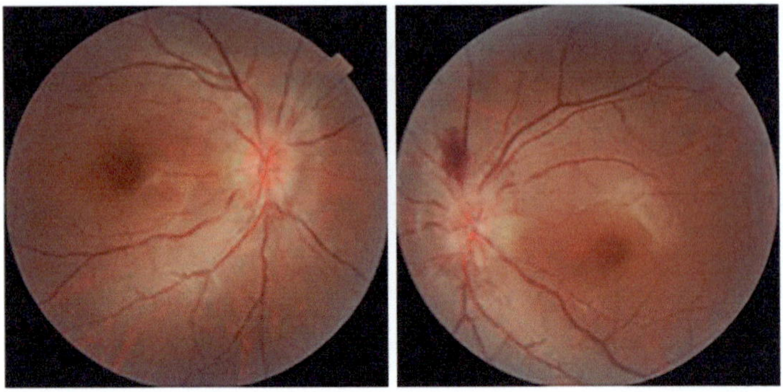

SIGNS

- Optic disc appearance:

Acute (weeks, months)
Normal (20-40%)
Hyperaemia, swelling, telangiectatic vessels, vascular tortuosity
Chronic (months, years)

- Atrophy, temporal pallor
- RAPD
- Reduced colour vision

Fig. 16.5 Leber's hereditary optic neuropathy

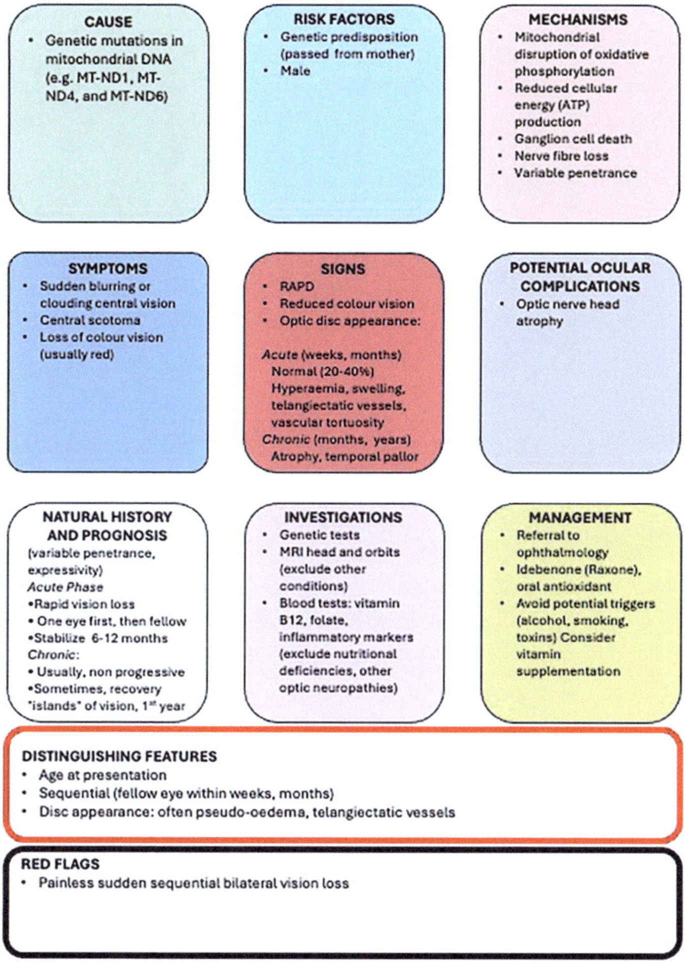

Fig. 16.6 Leber's hereditary optic neuropathy (illness script 47)

Table 16.1 Comparison of optic neuritis, anterior ischaemic optic neuropathy and Leber's hereditary optic neuropathy illness scripts

	Optic neuritis	Anterior ischaemic optic neuropathy	Leber's hereditary optic neuropathy
Cause	Inflammation Autoimmune (e.g. MS, NMO) Infections (e.g. mumps, Lyme disease, syphilis)	Ischaemia	Genetic mutations in mitochondrial DNA (e.g. MT-ND1, MT-ND4, and MT-ND6)
Risk factors	Female Aged 20–40 White ethnicity History of autoimmune disease Living farther from the equator Viral infections	Age (increased after 50) Diabetes Hypertension Hypercholesterolaemia Smoking Obstructive sleep apnoea Giant cell arteritis	Genetic predisposition passed on from the mother Variable penetrance More men than women develop symptoms
Mechanisms and pathogenesis	Autoimmune response Inflammation Trigger viral infection or MS or NMO Demyelination, conduction block Axonal damage	Ischemia (reduced optic nerve posterior ciliary arteries blood supply) Excitotoxicity Oxidative stress Apoptosis Retinal ganglion cell death Axonal degeneration	Mitochondrial disruption of oxidative phosphorylation Reduced cellular energy (ATP) production Ganglion cell death Nerve fibre loss

Symptoms	Sudden vision loss (mild to complete blur) Reduced colour vision (especially red) Visual field loss (central or peripheral) Flashing lights Heat-induced worsening of vision Often 1 eye (might be bilateral sequential) Pain (behind eye) worse with movement	Usually sudden vision loss (blurred, dim, blind spots) Reduced colour vision (washed out) Vision field defects Some cases eye pain	Sudden blurring or clouding central vision Central blind spot (scotoma) Severe visual loss Loss of colour vision (usually red)

(continued)

Table 16.1 (continued)

	Optic neuritis	Anterior ischaemic optic neuropathy	Leber's hereditary optic neuropathy
Signs	Reduced visual acuity (CF) Visual field defect: blind spot (scotoma) or peripheral vision Relative afferent pupillary defect Optic disc appearance	Reduced visual acuity (6/9-CF) Visual field defect (usually altitudinal) Relative afferent pupillary defect Optic disc appearance	Visual acuity RAPD Reduced colour vision Optic disc appearance: Acute stage (weeks to months) Normal (20–40%) Hyperaemia, swelling, telangiectatic vessels, vascular tortuosity: Chronic stage (months to years) Atrophy Temporal pallor (papillomacular bundle)
Complications	Optic atrophy Recurrences	Optic nerve atrophy Involvement of fellow eye	Optic nerve atrophy

Natural history and prognosis	Typically affects 1 eye but can affect both Sudden onset Worsen over hours-days Self-recovery over weeks to months (most close to normal, some remaining mild, permanent reduction) Recurrence: approximately 50% of MS patients within 5 years	Onset acute Recovery occasional, mild in non-arteritic (up to 40%) Permanent visual loss Fellow eye affected without treatment arteritic	Penetrance, expressivity and prognosis vary depending on the genetic mutation Acute Phase Rapid, painless vision Often starting in one eye first but affecting both Stabilization within 6–12 months Chronic phase: Vision loss is generally not progressive after acute phase but permanent Spontaneous recovery of small "islands" of vision might happen within the first year
Investigations	MRI head and orbit Blood tests (infections, aquaporin 4, MGO antibodies) Visual evoked potential (assessment optic pathway function) LP	BP Blood tests: cardiovascular risk factors, ESR, CRP	Genetic tests MRI head and orbits (exclude other conditions) Blood tests: B12, folate, inflammatory markers (exclude nutritional deficiencies, other optic neuropathies)

(continued)

Table 16.1 (continued)

	Optic neuritis	Anterior ischaemic optic neuropathy	Leber's hereditary optic neuropathy
Management	Referral to ophthalmology and/or neurology Observation (may improve spontaneously) Systemic steroids Plasma exchange Immunosuppressants for certain cases	Prompt systemic steroid treatment (arteritic, AION) Optimise cardiovascular risk factors Low vision aids	Referral to ophthalmology Idebenone (Raxone), oral antioxidant Avoid triggers (alcohol, smoking, toxins) Consider vitamin supplementation
Distinguishing features	Age at presentation Acute onset Pain with eye movement Recovery Recurrences Optic nerve inflammation seen on MRI Associated MS symptoms Often unilateral, may be sequential	Age at presentation Arteritic AION: elevated inflammatory markers (ESR, CRP), associated GCA symptoms Non arteritic ION: cardiovascular risk factors, normal inflammatory markers, no associated symptoms of GCA	Age at presentation Acute, subacute onset Painless Central vision loss Disc appearance: often pseudo-oedema, telangiectatic vessels Poor recovery Sequential (fellow eye within weeks, months)

Red flags	Bilateral simultaneously or sequential involvement Severe vision loss Slow prolonged loss Painless onset Poor steroid response Severe disc swelling (papilloedema) or haemorrhage, optociliary shunt vessels (suggesting compression)	GCA signs and/or symptoms (scalp tenderness, jaw claudication, pain, fatigue, PMR, general malaise) History of amaurosis fugax Rapidly sequential bilateral vision loss Elevated inflammatory markers	Painless sudden sequential bilateral vision loss

17 Thyroid Eye Disease, Periorbital and Orbital Cellulitis

Thyroid eye disease is an autoimmune condition that causes inflammation and swelling of the eye muscles and orbital tissues, often leading to symptoms like dry eyes, light sensitivity and proptosis, redness, swelling and double vision. It is most commonly associated with an overactive thyroid from Graves' disease but can also occur with an underactive or normal thyroid. While often mild, severe cases can threaten vision (Figs. 17.1 and 17.2). Periorbital (or preseptal) cellulitis is a superficial infection that progresses from the eyelid and tissues in front of the orbital septum (Figs. 17.3 and 17.4). Orbital cellulitis is a serious eye infection of the soft tissues and muscles within the orbit (behind the orbital septum) (Figs. 17.5 and 17.6).

The following illness scripts (Figs. 17.2, 17.4, and 17.6) and Table 17.1 compare the elements of thyroid eye disease, periorbital and orbital cellulitis, including distinguishing features and red flags.

M. Ugarte, *Ophthalmology Illness Scripts*,
https://doi.org/10.1007/978-3-032-31008-8_17

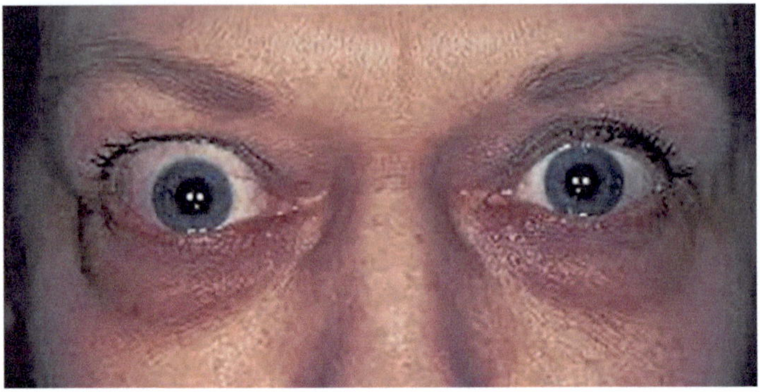

SIGNS

- Chemosis
- Proptosis
- Eyelid retraction
- Dry cornea
- Restriction of eye movements

Fig. 17.1 Thyroid eye disease

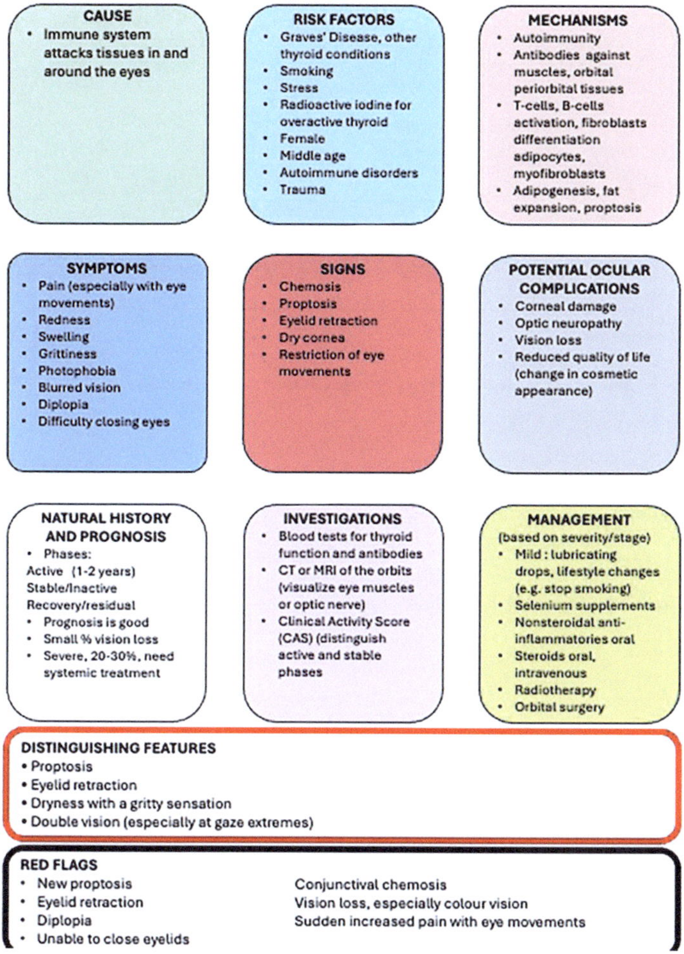

Fig. 17.2 Thyroid eye disease illness script (illness script 48)

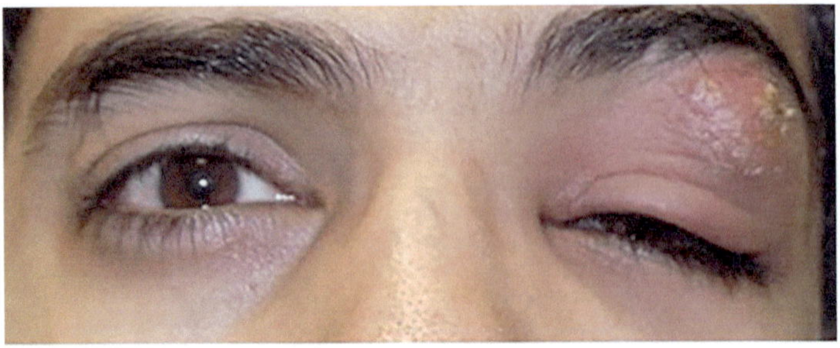

SIGNS

- Swollen, red, tender eyelids
- Swollen, red, tender surrounding soft tissues (anterior to orbital septum)

Fig. 17.3 Periorbital cellulitis

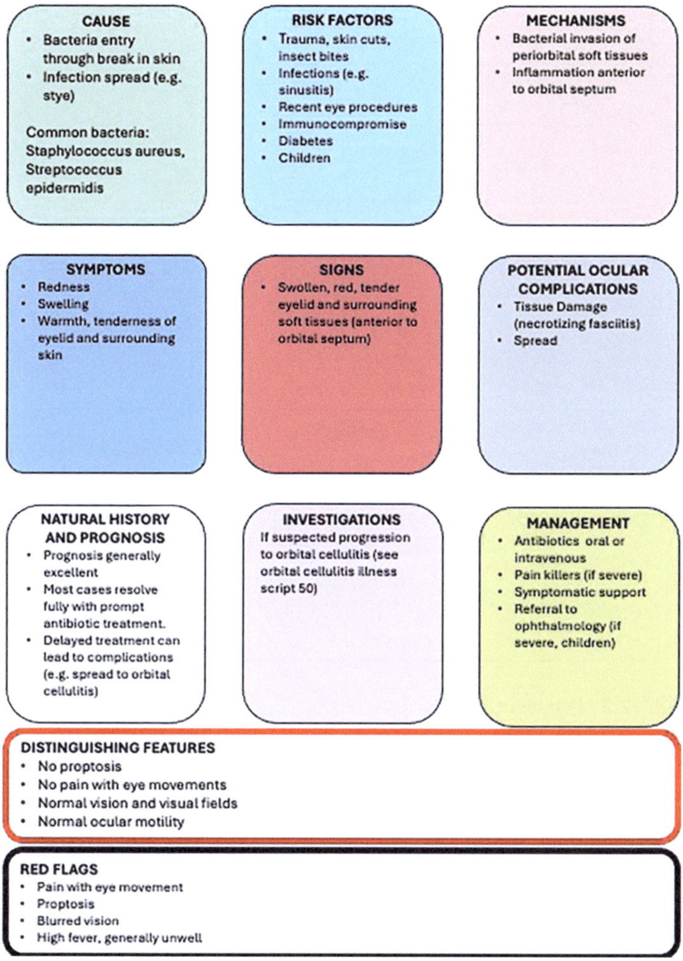

Fig. 17.4 Periorbital cellulitis illness script (illness script 49)

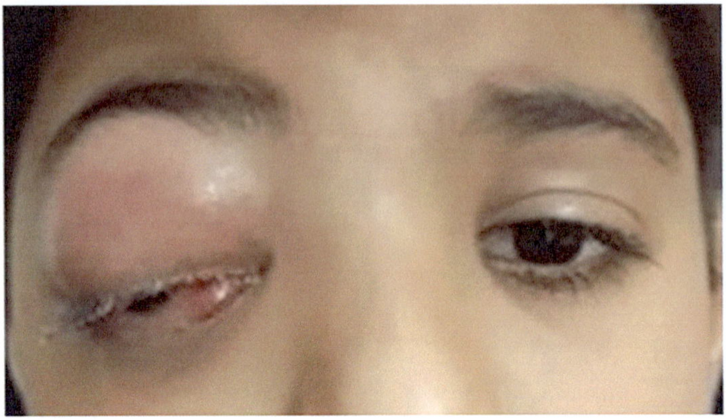

SIGNS

- Proptosis
- Redness
- Chemosis
- Discharge

Fig. 17.5 Orbital cellulitis

CAUSE
- Infection spreading from nearby areas, commonly sinuses also from eyelid

Common bacteria: Staphylococcus aureus, Streptococcus pyogenes, Haemophilus influenzae

RISK FACTORS
- Children
- Recent cold, sore throat, sinusitis
- Recent eye trauma, bite, sting, surgery, foreign body
- Diabetes
- Immunocompromise

MECHANISMS
- Direct or venous spread
- Inflammation and oedema
- Infection orbital tissues behind orbital septum

SYMPTOMS
- Swelling
- Redness
- Difficulty opening the eye
- Pain with eye movement
- Decreased vision
- Diplopia
- Fever
- Generally unwell

SIGNS
- Proptosis
- Redness
- Chemosis
- Discharge

POTENTIAL OCULAR COMPLICATIONS

Vision loss
Optic nerve damage
Spread from orbit (meningitis, brain abscesses, cavernous sinus thrombosis)

)

NATURAL HISTORY AND PROGNOSIS
- Good prognosis with prompt diagnosis and antimicrobial treatment
- Delayed treatment, potential permanent vision loss, intracranial infections, even death

INVESTIGATIONS
- CT head scan with contrast
- MRI
- Swabs from any wounds or discharge
- Lumbar puncture (if suspected CNS involvement)
- Blood Tests: FBC, cultures, ESR, CRP

MANAGEMENT
- Hospitalization
- Intravenous antibiotics. Referral to ophthalmology and ENT
- Surgery, drainage may be necessary for abscess
- Supportive care
- Cool compresses

DISTINGUISHING FEATURES
- Proptosis
- Restricted eye movements
- Chemosis
- Visual impairment

RED FLAGS
- Diplopia
- Pain with eye movements
- Fever, malaise, headache

Fig. 17.6 Orbital cellulitis illness script (illness script 50)

Table 17.1 Comparison of thyroid eye disease, orbital and periorbital cellulitis illness scripts

	Thyroid eye disease	Orbital cellulitis	Periorbital cellulitis
Cause	Immune system attacks tissues in and around the eyes	Infection spreading from nearby areas, most commonly the sinuses (ethmoid/frontal), but also from eyelid chalazion, ears or blood Common bacteria: *Staphylococcus aureus*, *Streptococcus pyogenes*, *Haemophilus influenzae*	Bacteria entering through a break in the skin (e.g. insect bites, cuts, or facial trauma) Infections spreading from nearby areas like eyelid chalazion Common bacteria: *Staphylococcus aureus* and *Streptococcus epidermidis*
Risk factors	Graves' disease, other thyroid conditions Smoking Stress Radioactive iodine for overactive thyroid Female Middle age Autoimmune disorders Trauma	Children Recent cold, sore throat, or sinus issues Recent eye injury, bite, or sting or surgery Underlying conditions (e.g. diabetes) Immunocompromised Trauma Foreign bodies	Skin breaches (trauma, cuts, insect bites), nearby infections (sinusitis, eyelid, ear/face), recent eye procedures Immunocompromised Diabetes Children

Mechanisms	Autoimmunity Antibodies target muscles, fat tissue orbital and periorbital T cells and B cells orchestrate and maintain the autoimmune process Inflammation Activated orbital fibroblasts differentiate into adipocytes and myofibroblasts Production of pro-inflammatory cytokines, chemokines and hyaluronan Adipogenesis Orbital fat expansion and proptosis	Direct or venous spread Infection orbital fat and muscles behind the orbital septum Inflammation and oedema	Bacterial invasion of periorbital soft tissues Inflammation and swelling anterior to orbital septum
Symptoms	Pain (especially with eye movements) Redness Swollen Gritty, dry Sometimes watery Photophobia Blurred vision Diplopia Difficulty closing the eyes	Eyelid swelling Redness Difficulty opening the eye Pain with eye movement Decreased vision Diplopia Fever General illness	Redness Swelling Warmth, tenderness of eyelid and surrounding skin Fever Generally unwell

(continued)

Table 17.1 (continued)

	Thyroid eye disease	Orbital cellulitis	Periorbital cellulitis
Signs	Chemosis Proptosis Eyelid retraction Dry cornea Restriction of eye movements	Proptosis	Swollen, red and tender eyelid
Complications	Corneal damage Optic neuropathy Vision loss Quality of life (cosmetic appearance)	Vision loss Optic nerve damage Meningitis Brain abscesses Cavernous sinus thrombosis	Permanent vision impairment or blindness Intracranial spread: meningitis, brain abscess, or cavernous sinus thrombosis (blood clot in brain sinus) Tissue damage (necrotizing fasciitis)

Natural history	Active phase (typically 6–24 months) Stable/inactive phase: inflammation subsides, symptoms stabilize, fibrotic stage with tissue scarring Recovery/residual phase: improvement happens, but often some scarring remains Prognosis is generally good Most people have mild symptoms that often resolve spontaneously Small percentage vision loss Severe cases: up to 20–30% need anti-inflammatory treatment (like steroids)	Uncomplicated cases show improvement within 24–48 h of treatment More severe cases, good prognosis with prompt diagnosis and timely intravenous antibiotics (full recovery with no lasting complications in most cases) Delayed treatment can lead to severe outcomes, including permanent vision loss, intracranial infections and potential death	Prognosis is generally excellent, most cases resolve fully with prompt antibiotic treatment Delayed treatment can lead to complications such as orbital cellulitis, vision loss, intracranial infections like meningitis or cavernous sinus thrombosis

(continued)

Table 17.1 (continued)

	Thyroid eye disease	Orbital cellulitis	Periorbital cellulitis
Investigations	Clinical eye examinations (assessment of visual acuity, visual fields, eye movements, eyelid position, proptosis) Blood tests for thyroid function and antibodies CT or MRI of the orbits (visualize eye muscles or optic nerve) Clinical activity score (distinguish active and stable phases by grading classic signs of inflammation)	CT scan with contrast to confirm diagnosis, determine location and presence of abscess MRI (superior soft tissue detail) Swabs from any wounds or discharge Potentially lumbar puncture if CNS involvement is suspected Blood tests: FBC, cultures, ESR, CRP	CT scan with contrast to confirm diagnosis, determine location, abscess presence/absence MRI (superior soft tissue detail) Swabs from any wounds or discharge Potentially LP if CNS involvement suspected Blood tests: FBC, cultures, ESR, CRP

Management	Depends on severity and stage Mild cases: lubricating eye drops Lifestyle changes like stopping smoking Selenium supplements: may help Active, severe cases: Intravenous or oral steroids Severe active cases, radiation therapy Surgery: correct lid position or eye muscle alignment. Rehabilitative surgery, such as orbital decompression or eye muscle surgery, can correct eye protrusion, nerve compression, and double vision once inflammation has settled Oral nonsteroidal anti-inflammatory drugs	Hospitalization Referral to ophthalmology and ENT Intravenous antibioticsbroad-spectrum coverage. Step-down therapy after clinical improvement. Switch to oral (e.g., co-amoxiclav) to complete course 7–10 days for uncomplicated cases, but can extend to 2–4 weeks for severe infections Surgery, drainage may be necessary for abscess identified on the CT scan or if the infection is not responding to antibiotics Supportive care: elevating the head with pillows can help reduce swelling Cool compresses	Oral or intravenous (IV) antibiotics to treat the bacterial infection, depending on severity Broad spectrum to cover bacteria like *Staphylococcus aureus*, Streptococcus species, and anaerobes Pain management: Symptomatic support: Referral and monitoring: Ophthalmology/ENT review

(continued)

Table 17.1 (continued)

	Thyroid eye disease	Orbital cellulitis	Periorbital cellulitis
Distinguishing features	Proptosis Eyelid retraction Dryness with a gritty sensation Double vision (especially at gaze extremes)	Proptosis Pain with eye movements Restricted eye movement Vision impairment Chemoses RAPD	No proptosis No pain with eye movements Normal vision and visual fields Normal ocular motility
Red flags	New proptosis Eyelid retraction Vision loss, especially colour vision Diplopia Sudden pain in or behind the eyes, particularly with eye movements Eyelid swollen, red, unable to close Conjunctival chemosis Dryness, excessive watering, photophobia	Pain with eye movements Proptosis Decreased vision Loss of colour vision Restricted eye movements Swelling, and redness of the eye and surrounding tissues Fever Malaise Headache Pupil abnormalities	Pain with eye movement Proptosis Blurred vision Reduced colour vision Abnormal pupil reactions Restricted eye movement High fever Generally unwell Lack of improvement on oral antibiotics

Appendix A: Practise Your Clinical Reasoning Using Illness Scripts (Red Eye) (see Fig. A.1)

M. Ugarte, *Ophthalmology Illness Scripts*,
https://doi.org/10.1007/978-3-032-31008-8

	Your patient	Conjunctivitis	Keratitis	Anterior uveitis	Episcleritis	Scleritis	Acute glaucoma
Cause							
Risk factors							
Mechanisms and pathogenesis							
Symptoms							
Signs							
Complications							
Natural history and prognosis							
Investigations							
Management							
Distinguishing features							
Red flags							

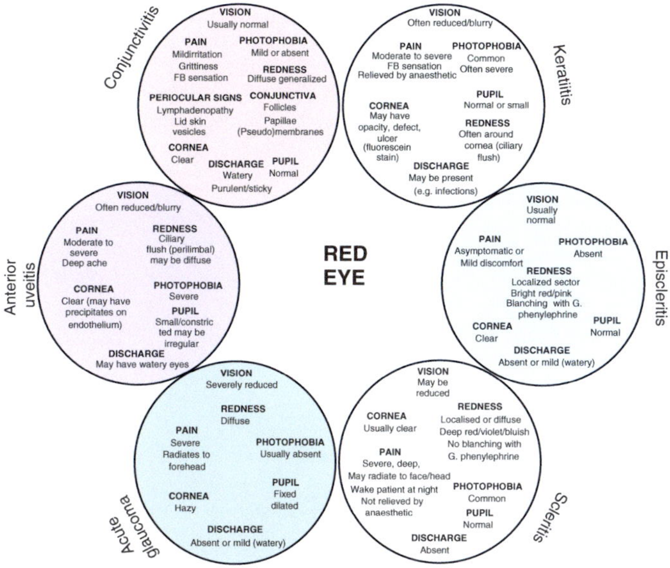

Fig. A.1 Distinguishing features of conditions causing red eye

FSC
www.fsc.org

MIX
Papier aus verantwortungsvollen Quellen
Paper from responsible sources
FSC® C105338

If you have any concerns about our products,
you can contact us on
ProductSafety@springernature.com

In case Publisher is established outside the EU,
the EU authorized representative is:
Springer Nature Customer Service Center GmbH
Europaplatz 3, 69115 Heidelberg, Germany

Printed by Libri Plureos GmbH
in Hamburg, Germany